Let Me Tell You
a Story

Inspirational Stories
for Health, Happiness,
and a Sexy Waist

James O'Keefe, MD, with Joan O'Keefe, RD

D1469104

Andrews McMeel
Publishing, LLC
Kansas City · Sydney · London

Andrews McMeel Publishing, LLC
an Andrews McMeel Universal company
1130 Walnut Street, Kansas City, Missouri 64106

www.andrewsmcmeel.com

13 14 15 16 17 MLT 10 9 8 7 6 5 4 3 2 1

ISBN: 978-1-4494-0777-3
Library of Congress Control Number: 2013930147

Cover Design: Zachary Cole
Cover Photography: Judy Williams
Editor and Interior Design: Rebecca M. Korphage
Cover Model: Kathleen O'Keefe

Disclaimer
The information in this book, including discussions of diet, exercise and fitness regimens, supplements, and medications, is intended to be used for educational purposes only. This book should not be used as a guide to diagnose and/or treat medical illnesses. The authors and publisher specifically disclaim any and all liability arising from the use or application of the information contained within this book. Before beginning a diet and exercise program, we recommend that you consult with a health care professional.

ATTENTION: SCHOOLS AND BUSINESSES
Andrews McMeel books are available at quantity discounts with bulk purchase for educational, business, or sales promotional use. For information, please e-mail the Andrews McMeel Publishing Special Sales Department: specialsales@amuniversal.com

DEDICATION

We dedicate this book to our children,
Jimmy, Evan, Kathleen, and Caroline.

CONTENTS

Part II

ACKNOWLEDGMENTS

We would like to acknowledge all of the characters (people and animals) depicted in these stories. Being allowed to share in their experiences, and then integrating those insights with cutting edge science is the essence of this book. Our combined expertise in the fields of cardiology and nutrition, and our driving passion for health and well-being have given us an ability to interpret these moments and weave them into a tapestry from which emerges a clear and beautiful picture. Our fondest wish is that these characters, whom we love dearly, will help you become the picture of health.

PREFACE

The Power of a Story

We have 4 children; I have been telling them bedtime stories for 26 years. Our youngest child, Caroline, just turned 13 and my bedtime story telling days are winding down. Still, people of all ages love to hear stories; they entertain us, but they also teach us about the world. Joan often speaks on nutrition, and loves how, when she says, "Let me tell you a story," the audience sets down their smart phones and reading materials, looks intently up at her and listens in rapt attention. Story telling is not only fun but also is how the human brain best learns new concepts and internalizes information that can change one's perspective and alter behavior.

We are all immersed in 'data-smog' today. Scientific findings and statistics are churned out at an ever-quickening pace. Recent estimates state that the entire body of scientific knowledge has doubled just since the year 2000. It has become unmanageable to keep up with all the science on health, nutrition, fitness, and wellness. So many people just throw up their hands in frustration, not knowing what to believe, while continuing to follow lifestyles and diets that are often toxic. Yet knowledge is power; you and your loved ones need this information if you are to thrive in this 21st century environment that is so foreign to our genetic identity.

This is a book of true stories about real people, though their names have been changed except where they have preferred that we disclose their identities. The stories might be derided as anecdotal by hardcore scientists, but we used them as examples to illustrate important concepts based on state-of-the-art science and the power of our Forever Young Diet and Lifestyle program (as we outlined in our previous book by the same title).

Story telling is as old as the human race. A story is the retelling of an experience, described with enough detail and feeling to make it seem real to the reader. We hope that these stories will inspire you to take advantage of the marvels of modern science, while at the same time remaining true to the diet and exercise patterns that bestowed strength and well-being upon our ancient ancestors while they were thriving in their wild, natural environment. Our driving passion is YOU. Your health, happiness, and longevity are deeply important to us: we hope you enjoy our stories, and that this book revolutionizes your life.

INTRODUCTION

Once Upon a Time...

A California girl with twinkling eyes and a charming smile met a guy in Minnesota who found her to be the most beautiful woman he had ever known. They fell in love, and after a couple years of dating they were married. One year later, at age 27, she became pregnant, which began innocently enough, but as the weeks ticked by her usual boundless energy started to diminish. By mid-pregnancy she felt drained, and her stamina was falling off dramatically. One cool April evening as they strolled together with his right arm draped around her shoulders, he happened to feel an ominous lump adjacent to her right collarbone. The next morning at her doctor's office, an X-ray confirmed their worst fears: a massive grapefruit-sized tumor was displacing her heart and lungs; the worrisome nodule they felt the day before was a metastasis. From there it was a downward spiral into a medical calamity and an emotional nightmare.

The doctors told them that the odds that the mother and her baby would both survive were small. The brightest and best cancer specialists at the Mayo Clinic urgently formulated a treatment to try to save the 2 of them from a large and aggressive malignancy that was on the move—its deadly tentacles invading throughout her chest. The jeopardized baby was to be protected from the radiation by a home-made wooden frame constructed in the garage of one of the X-ray technologists. Before each radiation therapy session this frame was positioned over her belly and then loaded sheet by sheet with 500 pounds of lead. Nearly lethal doses of radiation were focused at the largest mass behind her breast-bone, while the tiny baby oblivious to the danger curled up in the womb only a few inches away from the targeted tumor. She received 8 weeks of daily radiation treatment, even as the baby inside her seemed to be growing normally.

The little family of 3 shuddered under the weight of their troubles—the lives of 2 of them hung in the balance. Already weakened by pregnancy, cancer, harsh radiation therapy, and severe anemia, she was now facing a major surgery to deliver the baby by Caesarian section and to remove her spleen. During the surgery, the C-section was performed first; once delivered, the premature baby turned blue as he struggled for oxygen. He was whisked away to the neonatal intensive care where he required emergency intubation and a ventilator to help him breathe. The mother came through the surgery, but still faced months more of radiation therapy in an attempt to fully eradicate the metastatic cancer.

> "My desire and my will were being driven by the love which moves the sun and the other stars."
> – From Dante's *Inferno*

This story might have ended badly, indeed the doctors told them to "Hope for the best but prepare for the worst." The morning after surgery, from her bed in the intensive care unit, the mother while staring at a Polaroid picture of her helpless and tiny newborn, tubes down his nose and mouth, a forlorn look in his eyes, felt a powerful force stirring within her soul. Moved by an intense and unstoppable love, she told herself during that moment "I **will** survive this siege, whatever it takes." She knew that her baby needed her desperately and that nobody could ever replace her maternal love and nurturing.

> "He who has a *why* to live, can bear almost any *how*."
> –Friedrich Nietzsche

The woman in this story is Joan, and the baby boy is our now 26-year-old son Jimmy (see back cover photo) who graduated from Harvard 4 years ago and is now enrolled in Harvard Business School. Incidentally, the other 3 kids in that photo on the back of the book are the natural-born children that the medical experts told Joan she would never have. This triumph against all odds was no coincidence. We learned how to take the best of both worlds: the wonders of modern medicine combined with healing and strength from following the natural diet and lifestyle of our ancient hunter-gatherer ancestors. Also, my wife and children might not be alive today if not for the support of our family, friends, and community who rallied behind us and buoyed our spirits during some dark days. And finally Joan's faith in God gave her the optimism and peace to endure and ultimately overcome a situation that would have otherwise felt overwhelming.

The experience transformed us in a baptism by fire, wherein we came to appreciate how precious life is, and how we need to take care of one another. I would like to tell you that this program is really complicated, and that we are really smart, but it's actually simple and straightforward. Part of our passion for longevity, health, and wellness comes from concern for our children. We want to help them to realize their full potential, live long and happy lives, and make the world a better place. **Your story** can be magical too, and we wrote this book for you.

PART I

CHAPTER 1

We're All in This Together

I am proud of the man for whom I was named. My father was better at connecting with people than anyone I've ever known. Born and raised in North Dakota, he came to view the entire state's population as his *tribe*. He was a judge for the State District Court and later the State Supreme Court. Whenever he met someone new, after just a few minutes of friendly conversation he would be able to find a shared acquaintance or interest. Nothing pleased him more than being able to weave someone into the tapestry of life that binds us all together and gives us a sense of shared identity and support.

With the lowest per capita crime rate in the U.S., the state motto of North Dakota could be "40 below zero keeps the riff-raff out." Indeed, about the only homeless person in our hometown of Grafton was an unfortunate man named Louie, who as insensitive kids, we nicknamed Screwy Louie. He was a gentle but tormented soul who suffered from paranoid schizophrenia. Louie lived in his jalopy of a car, fearing that if he moved into an apartment the state authorities would be able to track him down and lock him away in a mental ward. My father took Louie under his wing and found a heated bus barn in which Louie could park and live in his car and still stay warm during the frigid winters. My parents, for decades, paid Louie to shovel the snow from their sidewalks or mow the lawn; they treated him like family, and the 2 of them were the only people he trusted.

About 10 years ago, when my father suddenly fell ill, and was diagnosed with metastatic and terminal pancreatic cancer, Louie parked his car outside the small local hospital and wouldn't leave. For weeks, Louie, in his ragged, oil-stained parka, paced up and down the hospital's snowy sidewalks, muttering despondently under his breath. Late one night I happened upon Louie, cowering in a corner of the dimly lit, deserted hospital waiting room. In a frightened tone he pleaded, "You can't let your father die; I don't know what will become of me." Through tear-filled eyes I said, "Louie, we are all in this together; you will be ok." I hugged him and in that embrace I felt a bond of brotherhood that made a desperate time feel just a little more endurable for both of us.

The Only Thing That Really Matters

Since 1937, the Harvard Study of Adult Development has closely followed one entire class of Harvard students for more than 70 years, through college, careers, marriages, divorces, illnesses, and for many participants, even death. The study focused on how different behaviors are linked with various outcomes in terms of health, happiness, and longevity. According to writer Charles Wheelan, when the physician director of the Harvard Study was asked what this unique and comprehensive database revealed he replied, "The only thing that really matters in life are your relationships to other people." Truly, our interpersonal relationships dwarf every other factor in our lives for predicting the quality and quantity of our life. In other words family and friends are much, much more important to our physical and emotional well-being than money or anything else. For instance, recent studies show that belonging to a social group that meets even just once a month, has the same positive effect on your sense of well-being as doubling your income.

In his brilliant new book *Stresscraft* (an e-book available on amazon.com), my good friend Frank Forenich writes about how today's focus on the individual, rather than family, community, and tribe is unprecedented in human history. During the vast majority of human existence on Earth, people identified powerfully with their group. Ubuntu (pronounced oo-Boon'-too) is a traditional philosophy of the Bantu tribe from southern Africa that teaches that a connection exists between people, and it is through this bond that we discover our identity and our purpose in life. Ubuntu holds that, "I am what I am because of who we all are." The worldview of ubuntu speaks about belonging, about compassion, about being a valuable part of something bigger than each of us. In this way of life, when someone is degraded or humiliated, we are all diminished. According to Frank, "Ubuntu is not just idealistic Afro-hippie talk. It's solidly supported by the latest findings in social neuroscience and interpersonal neurobiology. The philosophy of ubuntu is practical, intelligent, and functional." This attitude that we all need each other gives us resilience, strength and assurance to persevere in the face of daunting hardships.

Louie's Home

After my father's death, Louie still stopped by my parents' house nearly every day to visit with my mother. Louie's paranoia mellowed a bit as he grew older and he allowed my mother and her friends Peggy and John to find him a government-subsidized apartment. He still wouldn't change his clothes, shower, or lay in the bed, but he discovered that sleeping on the couch was reassuringly similar to dozing off in the back seat of his car, except he stayed warm and comfortable all night long. One day Louie didn't stop by to check in with my mother, or John and Peggy. They found him in his apartment where he had passed away suddenly and quietly. For the majority of his nearly 80 years, Louie lived in the shadows of Grafton where his home was the street. Even so, through the decades he grew to be an integral resident and a beloved character. The townspeople turned out in droves for his funeral, and they mourned for Louie as if he was one of their own family.

Oxytocin: The Goodness We Seek

Paul Zak is a renowned researcher who has spent his career studying the hormone oxytocin. In his new book, *The Moral Molecule*, Zak explains that empathic human connection stimulates oxytocin release in the brain, which in turn engenders trust and affection, forges interpersonal bonds, inspires altruism and generosity, and is the hormonal basis for love and prosperity. Each of us has the capacity to be both good and bad, depending on the circumstances and influences in our lives. In stable and safe surroundings, oxytocin makes us generally good, and leads to loyalty, generosity, and cooperation. He calls testosterone oxytocin's evil twin; high levels of testosterone cause a hell of a lot of trouble, and not just for interpersonal relationships. For instance, most violent crimes are committed by young men, generally between the ages of 18 and 25, when testosterone levels tend to be through the ceiling. On the other hand high oxytocin levels are all good—for example, childbirth and nursing an infant stimulate sky-high oxytocin levels which instill the intense, fierce maternal love that one could argue might be the most powerful force in nature, for without it mammalian life would not flourish or even survive. In response to all varieties of stimuli, women typically make a lot more of this hormone than men, which I believe at least in part explains why women tend to outlive men by about 5 years. Studies show that higher oxytocin levels inspire us to be not only generous and kind, but also have a greater sense of security and more satisfaction with life, better resilience to setbacks, higher quality relationships, closer family ties, and more friends.

Channeling the Better Angels of Our Nature

So why can't we just take an oxytocin pill every morning to make our life wonderful? If only it were that simple. This hormone lasts only a few minutes in the bloodstream, so if you want high levels, you need to earn them the old-fashioned way—by stimulating your pituitary gland to make more of the good stuff. Zak, who has been dubbed "Dr. Love," writes that his prescription for increasing one's oxytocin levels is to play with your kids, have fun and emotionally bond with your friends, hold hands, give and get massages, kiss and have more sex with your significant other, join social groups, get a dog, and follow the "Golden Rule"—treat others as you would want to be treated. And one more practical tip: each day try to give at least 8 hugs (all to 1 person or to 8 different people, whatever works for you). Zak and his colleagues have shown that if you give 8 hugs daily you will be happier. This kind of behavior can create a virtuous cycle whereby altruism and caring for others stimulates oxytocin, and higher levels of this hormone inspire us and the people with whom we are interacting to be more trusting, loyal, and loving. This positive feedback loop sends ripples of trust and affection out into your world, making it a kinder and gentler place in which to live.

My instincts tell me hugging your dog or cat works just as well as hugging a person, but hugging a tree... maybe not so much. I must admit, when I was younger, I used to be a bit embarrassed when a patient would hug me; but these days a hug never fails to warm my heart and make me smile.

Traveling Light Through Life

After graduating from college our oldest son Jimmy and I packed all his belongings into a small rented truck and moved him across the country to start his first real job. When we arrived in New York City at 2:00 a.m., in the span of just 30 minutes, we carried all his possessions upstairs into a small yet functional apartment. It was an unforgettable adventure and it warmed my heart to see him, for the time being at least, unencumbered by all the material trappings that tend to accumulate in our modern culture. Jimmy walks or uses mass transit when he needs to go somewhere. He spends most of his free time and disposable income on enjoying life with his friends.

The Key to Life: More Experiences, Less Stuff

Who says you can't buy happiness? Turns out you can if you splurge on experiences instead of more stuff. Studies show that people who spend more of their discretionary income on interesting experiences rather than material things tend to be happier in the long run. Too much stuff, especially the expensive kind like extravagant houses, pricey motor vehicles, excessive wardrobes and jewelry, not only ensures that you have to put in the long hours at work to pay off those bills, but also turns your free time into more work time—as a maintenance person cleaning, fixing, protecting, worrying about, and insuring all those superfluous belongings. If you aren't careful, the materialistic frenzy created by American-style capitalism can lead you down a path where you find yourself feeling as though your possessions possess you, rather than the other way around.

Less Is More

Most of us already have more than enough stuff. Greed and envy are a waste of time and energy. I think we might all benefit from spending more of our time and money on experiences that make us happy, like fun vacations, a delicious and healthy meal out, music and concerts, exercise and fitness pursuits, or having a massage. Investing our time and energy into experiences, particularly those we can enjoy with our family and friends, is much more likely to enhance our lives in the long run than, say, another new car.

Of course not all the stuff you can buy is bad for you; a lovable dog, flowers for your sweetheart, comfortable walking shoes, are just a few exceptions that come to mind. Nor are all experiences you might choose to spend your money on (think cigarettes, video games, illicit drugs, prostitution...) good for your long-term health and happiness. Still, I try to remind myself that the consumerism promoted by 21st century life can sometimes turn into more of a shackle than a blessing. In my opinion, life is too short to drink bad wine, eat trashy food, and spend all my precious free time taking care of and worrying about stuff I don't really need.

Bringing Balance to Life

Many people notice that when they work too many hours, or too many days in a row, they start to get unhappy, cranky, and irritable. You may also notice that trying to focus on too many tasks at one time can leave you feeling nervous, numb, and overwhelmed. The conscious level of the human brain, amazing as it is, can only focus on a few things at once; and can only hold 1 thought at a time. So it is very important to prioritize the essential things in our lives.

A balanced life is a key to a healthy and happy heart, and vigorous longevity. We all get out of balance sometimes, and this creates stress in our lives and predisposes us to a sour attitude. On the other hand, balance feels good and promotes health, healing, and happiness. The more often you can achieve and maintain a healthy balance in your life, the better. Returning to the basics brings balance to our lives. Everyone has his or her own way of finding balance, but for most people it involves focusing on things like family and friends, rest and relaxation, fitness and fun, and nature and nutrition. You will find that if and when you make it a point to regularly devote time and energy to these priorities, you will feel more peaceful, less stressed, more energetic, and just happy to be alive, to use one of my mother's aphorisms. Especially when you are feeling stressed and under the gun, try to simplify your life by coming back to these fundamentals and see if restoring a healthy balance doesn't help to make your heart feel more at peace.

Between the Devil and Deep Blue Sea

The Boeing 767-400, with topped off fuel tanks and not a single empty seat, lumbered off the runway in Amsterdam bound for Chicago. Joan and I, on our way back home after a vacation in Europe, settled in with 250 other passengers, for what we expected to be an uneventful 9-hour-long flight. About 3 hours into the trans-Atlantic crossing, the pilot announced, in a tone that did not convey the confident reassurance that one comes to expect from an airliner captain, "We have a medical emergency. If there is a medical doctor on board, please report to the back of the plane." Joan looked at me, raised her eyebrows and then glanced back over her shoulder. I quickly made my way to the back of the cabin to find a very pale, cold and clammy, middle-aged man in severe distress who looked as though he was about to lose consciousness. I had him lie down on the floor immediately, and found out that he was a Dutchman named Johan who felt somewhat unwell before boarding the plane. As we ventured out across the wide ocean, he was now clutching his belly and complaining of "the worst pain in his life." I quickly examined him, and though I just barely touched his abdomen, he writhed in agony, pushing my hands away. His belly was as tight as a drum, and as I listened with a stethoscope, I heard no bowel sounds. Johan had an acute abdomen, which is a potentially life-threatening emergency, often necessitating urgent surgery. Except we were thousands of miles away from the nearest hospital, and Johan was looking shocky, with pulse of 110 and a blood pressure of only 70/40. I placed an intravenous line and administered fluids, but had no other therapies with which to treat him; specifically, the emergency medical kit contained no morphine or antibiotics. I did my best to comfort Johan, but both he and I understood the unspoken reality—we were between the Devil and deep blue sea.

I discussed our predicament with the captain over the phone, and he explained that we could circle back to Iceland or forge ahead to northeastern Canada, but either option was about 3 hours away. I told him that wherever we land, we would need an ambulance waiting, and a nearby hospital. A moment later, we heard the engines roar to full-throttle as the plane's nose tipped upward—climbing to a higher altitude that would allow for faster speeds. We hurtled towards North America and Johan soldiered on, patiently and silently enduring the ordeal, as I knelt on the galley floor next to him. Though the intravenous fluids had stabilized his blood pressure, the bag was nearly empty, his pain was worsening again, and now he was also developing shaking chills. The thought occurred to me that maybe this was an example of Einstein's Theory of Relativity: the faster we flew, the slower time seemed to be moving.

After what felt like an eternity, we approached our destination, Goose Bay Airport. It is a remote airstrip surrounded on one side by the rocky Labrador coastline, and on the other 3 sides by hills densely forested with tall evergreens. Goose Bay, an airport built during World War II, was never designed to accommodate a fully loaded, modern jumbo-jet airliner. In fact, the runway was about 30 percent shorter than what was usually required for a jet of this size. Blustery winds from a Nor'easter were howling off the Atlantic Ocean, and as we circled overhead, the captain jettisoned fuel to drop some weight from the plane to make the landing safer. The plane pitched wildly as the captain fought the cross winds and finally broke through a very low cloud ceiling. He set the 767 down hard on the tarmac and slammed on the brakes.

We offloaded Johan by stretcher into a 1960s vintage model ambulance, and I gave report to a local paramedic who spoke in a strange thick Scottish-sounding dialect that was barely recognizable as English. I laid one hand on Johan's shoulder, and with the other I gently squeezed his hand and told him that he was stable and that a physician was waiting for him just up the road at an emergency room. He looked up at me as his eyes welled up and said, "Thank you, doctor." I scampered up the stairs to the plane and stood there watching the ambulance pull away, bound for the little hospital in Happy Valley. I turned to notice that the sun was already setting—at about 4 in the afternoon. After the plane was refueled and de-iced, we sat at one end of the airstrip, waiting for what seemed to be a very long time. When we did take off, I looked down and saw the runway disappear from under our wings just a few seconds after we were airborne. I was guessing that the captain's blood pressure at that moment was at the other end of the spectrum from Johan's—probably about 180/95.

I heard from Johan a few days later. He had a large kidney stone blocking the flow from 1 kidney, resulting in so much pain and inflammation that it also caused a bowel obstruction. After a surgical procedure, he was recovering well, and was expecting to be discharged from the hospital soon. The episode reminded me how grateful I am to be in a healing profession; the opportunity to make a positive difference for a person in trouble is by far the most rewarding part of my job. You might make a living from what you get, but I think you make a life by what you give.

CHAPTER 2

The Magic in Your Genes

As scientists continue to unlock the secrets encoded within our genes, the implications for curing disease and extending life expectancy will make today's high-tech therapies look old-fashioned. Cures, not just temporary treatments, will be bio-engineered for obesity, diabetes, many cancers, high blood pressure, and even baldness, to name just a few breakthroughs on the horizon. But the dawning of that era is still at least 5 to 10 years away, so for today, you are stuck with the genes you inherited from your parents at the moment of your conception. Yet, we are discovering that your genes do not lock you into a biological destiny. True, your DNA starts out as 'hard-wired,' but even in the womb your genes respond dramatically to their environment. This chapter is about how you can influence your genetic expression and DNA function by altering your diet, lifestyle, attitudes, and habits so as to turn on genes for vitality and turn off genes that predispose to aging and disease. In this way you can rebuild a stronger, healthier, even genetically younger you just by changing the signals you send your genes.

Rejuvenate Your Life by Activating Your Genes

In your genes (I am not referring to your Levi's) did you know you have DNA lying dormant that, when activated, can rejuvenate your body and reinvigorate your life? Nature equipped you before you were born with a set of unimaginably complex and intelligent instructions in the form of DNA. Contained within this blueprint is everything you need to take your body and mind to new levels of vitality and health.

All of your ancient ancestors had one thing in common—they survived daunting threats (at least long enough to have children) and overcame obstacles and hardships in the wild and natural world. Your DNA is a legacy passed down to you from thousands of generations of the fittest individuals. You have the best of their collective genes, all meticulously spelled out within the DNA of your genome. Yet many of these genes lay inactive, waiting for you to awaken them by following the natural diet, lifestyle, and attitudes that confer the robust health, resiliency, and youthful vigor that made it possible for your ancestors to survive and thrive while living in the wild.

Yours is a bloodline of courageous souls who conquered tough times by growing tougher themselves. Their hardiness lives on in you, but you will never see it fully manifest while just coasting along on the path of least effort. No, if you want to grow stronger, you will have to exert yourself physically, like your ancestors were forced to do in order to endure their day-to-day rigors. And if you want to become lean, tough, and resilient, you will have to consume fewer calories by avoiding processed foods and instead eat, almost exclusively, highly nutritious natural, real foods. Finally, you have to avoid the victim mentality, and exchange any passive, self-obsessed, depressed, pessimistic, and fatalistic attitudes for a more hopeful, optimistic, can-do, community-minded, upbeat, and energetic outlook. Don't settle for a life of dragging around feeling helpless, tired, broken, weak, ill, or overwhelmed. Unbeknownst to you, deep within your being you already have what it takes to restore vibrant health and well-being. This genetic destiny can crystallize into reality when you immerse yourself in conditions that more closely simulate the diet, exercise and social settings of your ancient ancestors as they lived in the wilderness, in harmony with the natural world. Through your actions and attitudes, you can speak to those genes lying dormant within you and call forth the DNA that codes for natural strength, beauty, and heartiness.

"How many healthy people do you know?
How many happy people do you know? Think about it.
People work at dying, they don't work at living.
My workout is my obligation to life."
–Jack LaLanne

A cactus struggling to survive in the mild and rainy climate with rich and fertile soil in a Pacific Northwest rainforest will wilt and grow weak and sickly. And while you might be able to keep it alive with special plant food and grow lights, if you want it to really flourish, all you have to do is transplant it back to its native Sonoran Desert in Arizona. This arid region with its intense sunlight is a harsh climate that would kill most life, but because these are the conditions for which it is genetically designed, the cactus not only survives, it thrives. This environment resonates with the cactus's genetic identity, thereby booting up dormant genes. Soon the plant will regain its luster, resiliency, and vitality as it blossoms again in its natural home. Nothing in the world will revitalize a life form—plant or animal—as well as re-immersing it in its natural environment and diet.

Like the cactus, each one of us has powers of self-healing and renewal lying latent within our chromosomes. You are living in an unnatural world under conditions that are foreign to your genetic heritage and this bewilders your genes and causes them to malfunction. A cushy, inactive lifestyle with a glut of nutritionally barren calories signals our genes to lapse into the decay mode, predisposing to lethargy and disease. Rich, high-calorie foods and temporary reprieves from strenuous physical work were rare and unexpected windfalls for our ancestors. Now, these luxurious conditions, which were once uncommon treats, dominate the day-to-day life of most Americans. As a species, we have had insufficient time to genetically adapt to these modern affluent living conditions, sometimes referred to as *affluenza*. As a result, most people have difficulty resisting their instincts to eat too much and exercise too little, let alone physically cope with the destructive health effects of these behaviors. To be sure, we, the overfed citizens of this ultra-convenient 21st century culture, are becoming victims of our own success.

> ## "Life begins outside your comfort zone."
> –Mark Freed, M.D.

Get out of your comfort zone and start challenging yourself by reconnecting with the natural world; this is the surest way to automatically revitalize your health. When you engage in a lifestyle that includes vigorous physical activity and fresh air, naturally nutritious, low-calorie whole foods, and an attitude of optimism, belonging, and purpose, those previously dormant and quiescent genes will revive and reboot. These are the conditions that signal your genes that spring has arrived on the savannah, and it is time to kick-start your cells back into the thrive mode, which quickly leads to growth and regeneration.

Exercise has a particularly potent effect on activating these hibernating genes that can rejuvenate your mind and body. A moderate dose of daily physical exertion has been estimated to substantially change the function of almost half of the 20,000 genes in the human genome. This means that a consistent regimen of just 30 to 50 minutes of daily exercise will literally rebuild a whole new you. You have far more strength and resiliency within you than you realize. You have been pre-programmed to be able to rise to new levels of strength, vitality, and health. You can rebuild yourself from the inside out by channeling your ancient ancestors and reactivating the genes that will allow you to become the very best you can be.

"I am the grain of sand, becoming a pearl."
–Paula Cole

Steps That Activate Your Genes for Rejuvenation

1. <u>Challenge yourself through daily exercise</u>. Make sure you cross-train by doing a variety of activities, including cardio, strength exercises, and some stretching. Do some interval training which involves intermittent, short bursts of higher intensity exercise, with rest or lower intensity activity as you recover before the next interval.

2. <u>Rest your body</u>. After exercising hard, let your body rest, recover, and rebuild. Shoot for 7½ to 9 hours of sleep each 24-hour period. Nap 30 minutes as needed and when possible.

3. <u>Stay sexually active</u>. Make sure to practice safe sex, ideally at least 2 or 3 times weekly with your significant other.

4. <u>Cut down on your calorie intake</u>. Eat a diet that is rich in plants such as fresh and/or frozen vegetables and fruits, as well as nuts; also consume plenty of lean protein; and drink green tea, coffee, and water.

5. <u>Eat whole, natural foods</u>. Avoid processed foods, and almost everything that has more than 3 ingredients in the 'ingredients list.'

6. <u>Reduce your salt intake</u>. Your salt intake should be less than 2,300 mg daily. Almost 90 percent of the salt you eat is in the form of processed foods, typically the other 10 percent is added using a salt shaker.

7. <u>Increase fiber consumption</u>. Aim for 30 to 44 or more grams of fiber daily. Vegetables and fruits are the best way to get fiber.

8. <u>Have fun</u>. Invest more time and positive energy in your family, friends, pets, and gardens or hobbies.

9. <u>Enjoy nature</u>. Get outdoors every day for some fresh air. Try to get about 15 minutes of sunshine a day when possible.

10. <u>Think positively</u>. Try to frequently remind yourself of the various aspects of your life for which you are grateful. Visualize a more vigorous and youthful you. Believe that your best days are ahead.

Rebuilding a Whole New You from Your Genes Up

The body that you identify as *you* didn't exist a year ago. A living creature exists in a state of dynamic balance—with its cells, molecules, and atoms undergoing constant disposal and renewal. The collection of atoms and cells that manifest as your flesh, blood, bone, hair, eyes, teeth, etc., is completely different from one year to the next. Scientific studies performed at the Oak Ridge Atomic Research Center prove that 98 percent of all the atoms that make up a living human body are replaced each year. The cells in your skin are changed out once a month; your liver in just 6 weeks; the lining of your GI tract from your mouth, esophagus, stomach, and all the way to the end of your intestines lasts a mere 5 days before it is replaced. Even your bones are not the rock-like foundation you imagine them to be. They are undergoing continual breakdown and rebuilding, and are completely renewed within 1 year's time. In fact, 100 percent of the atoms in your body undergo a complete turnover within 5 years or less.

The collective genetic code of the human population, however, changes only 0.1 percent every 10,000 years. In other words, if the 20,000 genes in our genome were a deck of cards, they simply get reshuffled for every new individual; but the genes themselves are not altered significantly from generation to generation. However, the way the genes are expressed is highly influenced by the environment around us. A single gene can make hundreds or thousands of different proteins, thereby creating vastly differing effects for an individual. The rapidly evolving science of how genes are turned on and off is called *epigenetics*. Through an unimaginably complex and nuanced process, epigenetics exerts its astonishing intelligence and foresight. As we are coming to understand, the most important feature of our genome may be its plasticity and malleability; your gene expression, that is, how different segments of the DNA gets turned on or off, is almost 90 percent determined by the environment in which we are immersed. And that environment (our diet, lifestyle, social interactions, etc.) has changed more in the last century than in all of the previous 150,000-year human existence. In other words, your genes may load the gun, but your environment pulls the trigger.

Because your body is always in a state of flux, it is possible to re-create a whole new you by focusing on turning on the genes for youthful vigor and good health, and turning off the bad genes that code for degeneration and disease. Optimizing your genome—the instruction book from which your body continually renews and rebuilds itself—is the key to revitalizing your health. If you want to stay youthful and strong, you need to keep your DNA in pristine condition which will prevent entropy, the universal tendency for order to degenerate into disorder, from ravaging your body and brain.

Shut Down Premature Aging

Just 2 months after our son Evan was born, we brought home a cute little 8-week-old golden retriever puppy named Lacy. At their one-year birthday party Evan was still in diapers, couldn't walk or talk, and smeared chocolate cake all over his face as he tried to eat. Lacy, in contrast, sat regally next to him. She was already a smart and well-trained, 75-pound, full-grown adult. But as the years passed, Lacy began to grow old even though Evan was still growing up. She developed arthritis, cataracts, and bowel problems, slept more and more; and our irrepressibly good-natured Lacy sometimes got a bit grumpy. When she was 13, Lacy died of old age, while Evan was still waiting for the first signs of puberty to appear. Everything in the universe ages, even the universe itself will eventually die of old age (no worries—that's not expected for at least 100 trillion years). But how is it that the life cycle from birth to old age can be so different from one species to another? For example, a mouse becomes frail, demented, and arthritic before it celebrates its second birthday; while my grandmother Alice made it 93 years before she died of old age.

The rate of aging for living creatures is genetically determined, programmed by nature. But the pace of aging is in large part controlled by your genes themselves. Each of the 10 trillion cells that work together to make up your body has a full set of your DNA contained within chromosomes, which are X or Y-shaped structures. The ends of chromosomes are capped by telomeres, which are like the tips on the ends of shoelaces that keep them from fraying. Each time the cell divides to make a new copy of itself, the telomeres tend to grow shorter. So young individuals whether they are mice or humans, have long telomeres, and as an individual get older, his or her telomeres tend to shorten. When the telomere caps at the end of the chromosome are whittled away to nothing, the DNA unravels like a shoelace that has lost its plastic tip. In essence, once its telomere is used up, the cell can't make copies of itself anymore—which is a very, very big problem indeed, because a living creature that cannot regenerate new copies of the cells and tissues that are constantly being broken down will not be healthy or even alive for long.

Genetically Turning Back the Clock

You can dramatically change the rate that your telomere caps gets whittled away, and thus markedly slow the aging process and prevent many of the common diseases of old age. Astonishingly, by simply changing your diet and lifestyle, and taking a select few over-the-counter supplements, you can slow or stop the shortening of your telomeres and thus stay young much longer. Keeping your telomere caps long and intact and your DNA in its original, youthful condition will help to prevent age-related and inflammatory conditions that tend to accumulate like barnacles on the hull of a ship as the years and decades roll by. Everything from cancer, heart disease, vision loss from macular degeneration, arthritis, osteoporosis, and Alzheimer's disease might be prevented or markedly delayed by keeping one's telomeres intact.

Men tend to have shorter telomeres than women, probably because they burn through them faster by being more likely to engage in unhealthy, self-destructive behaviors (like smoking, poor diet, and excessive alcohol consumption). Women's slower telomere burn rate may in part explain why, on average, they live about 4 to 5 years longer than men.

In a recent study, men with low-grade prostate cancer were placed on a diet that eliminated processed carbohydrates, such as starches and refined sugars, and instead encouraged whole foods, especially vegetables, fruits, and berries. The men were also strongly advised to do daily moderate aerobic exercise, and practice relaxation techniques and breathing exercises. After 3 months on this regimen, participants were noted to have telomerase (an enzyme that prevents telomere shortening) levels that were 29 percent higher than their baseline levels. Another study showed that compared to men who didn't drink tea, men who drank 3 or more cups of tea daily had significantly longer telomeres, translating into a genetic age about 5 years younger than the non-tea drinkers.

Vitamin D Slows Telomere Aging

Vitamin D levels also appear to have an effect on telomere length. Studies indicate that restoring low vitamin D levels to normal reduces inflammation and slows the genetic aging process. Higher serum vitamin D concentrations are linked with significantly longer telomeres; this was equivalent to 5 years of additional lifespan. Ideal vitamin D levels are easily achieved via nutritional supplementation, and appear to help slow telomere loss and genetic aging. This may be part of the reason that low vitamin D levels are associated with many age-related diseases like cancer, diabetes, high blood pressure, osteoporosis, coronary artery disease, stroke, and neurodegenerative disorders such as Alzheimer's disease, multiple sclerosis, and Parkinson's disease.

Exercise for Preventing Genetic Aging

Studies in humans and animals consistently show that regular exercise is one of the best ways to slow telomere erosion and prevent premature genetic aging. Vigorous exercise, in particular, is associated with longer telomeres. Shorter telomere length has been suggested as an independent risk factor for cardiovascular disease.

Recently, a study evaluated the telomere length in young and middle-aged runners versus physically inactive (sedentary) people of similar ages. The sedentary middle-aged (mean age 51 years) subjects had telomeres that were 40 percent shorter compared with their sedentary younger (mean age 20 years) counterparts. In contrast, middle-aged runners had largely preserved their telomere length. Their telomeres were only 10 percent shorter than those of the young runners. In other words, long-term, high-level fitness as achieved by a regular running routine from age 20 to age 50 was associated with a 75 percent higher maintenance of telomere length, which translates to a much slower rate of aging.

Other studies have confirmed that maintaining a physically active lifestyle and high level fitness will confer an anti-aging effect. In fact, daily vigorous exercise has been shown to increase telomerase levels and slow telomere shortening in both humans and mice. Scientists have also noted that people and animals who maintain fitness over time also tend to even look and act younger than physically inactive individuals of the same age.

Stress and Aging

Have you ever noticed how some American presidents tend to age at hyper-speed while in office? One striking exception to this phenomenon was Harry Truman. He stayed hardy, healthy, and youthful despite taking over from FDR in 1945 during World War II. During his 8 years in office, and throughout his almost 90 years of life, Harry was a poster boy for healthy coping mechanisms.

Each morning he walked briskly, "As if I had some place important to be," as Harry liked to say. He also ate an almost ideal diet full of colorful fresh vegetables and fruits, and clean, unprocessed, natural protein sources—like fish and nuts. He had stress-relieving hobbies like playing the piano and socializing with family and friends, and he typically consumed just 1 alcoholic drink per day.

Scientific studies consistently show that high levels of emotional stress over time increase cardiovascular risk, impair immune function, worsen general health, and even shorten lifespan. The precise mechanisms by which chronic stress gets 'under our skin' remain somewhat unclear, but recent studies show that the cellular and genetic aging rate may play a role. Psychological stress has been linked with higher oxidative stress, and shorter telomere length. Shockingly, one study found that women with the highest levels of emotional stress had telomeres shorter on average by the equivalent of 1 decade of additional aging compared to low-stress women. In other words, a high-stress lifestyle can make you 10 years older than you really are. Importantly, in a recent study of women, those who reported high levels of emotional stress and were physically inactive had shorter telomeres; while a similar group of emotionally stressed women who exercised regularly show no accelerated shortening of their telomeres. To put it another way, uncontrolled stress can make you old before your time; fortunately, daily exercise seems to neutralize this stress-induced rapid aging. Our last 2 presidents, George W. Bush and Barack Obama, like "Give 'em Hell Harry," are regular exercisers, and they both also have seemed to hold up well physically under the unreasonable and unrelenting stress focused on an American President.

Omega-3 and Telomeres

The Japanese people on average live about 4 years longer than Americans, and have coronary heart disease rates less than half those found in the United States. Recent studies indicate that the "Japanese factor" responsible for their good health and longevity may be their high intake of fish, and more specifically the omega-3 fats present in seafood and fish.

Importantly, the average Japanese person consumes 5 to 8 times more fish than we do here in America. Two randomized controlled trials testing omega-3 fats, one in heart attack survivors and the other in patients with heart failure, showed that the purified fish oil significantly reduced death from *any cause*. Other studies suggest that omega-3 fats may help prevent Alzheimer's disease, macular degeneration, and coronary artery disease.

A recent study by Nobel Prize–winning scientist Elizabeth Blackburn showed that individuals who had blood omega-3 levels in the top 25 percent had a 70 percent reduction in the rate of telomere loss compared to those with low levels of omega-3. This means that omega-3 may delay genetic aging by slowing the telomere burn rate; and in so doing, may improve longevity and prevent age-related illnesses. Another study by Blackburn and colleagues was a randomized trial that found that an omega-3 daily supplement *lengthened* telomeres over a 4-month study period. An intake of 1,000 to 2,500 mg per day of omega-3 fats (DHA + EPA) from fish and/or fish oil is enough to get you into the level that bestows the protective effect on telomeres, improves longevity, and helps prevent the age-related illnesses like Alzheimer's disease and macular degeneration. This advice coincides nicely with the American Heart Association's recommendation of 1,000 mg a day of omega-3 fatty acids for the prevention of heart attack and stroke.

CHAPTER 3

Stress-Proof Your Life

"It is not the strongest of the species that survives, nor
the most intelligent that survives.
It is the one that is most adaptable to change."
–Charles Darwin

Too much stress can take the joy out of life and can ruin
your health. This chapter is about developing strategies to effectively deal with disruptive change and stress.

Bend Don't Break: How to Survive and Thrive in Times of Crisis and Upheaval

Paradoxically, change is the only thing in life of which we can
be certain. According to an old Chinese proverb, when the winds of
change blow, some people build walls, while others build windmills.
Flexibility of mind and body is a defining characteristic of youth.
Still, with focus and effort you can continue to be open-minded and
adaptable no matter what your age. It is especially during times of
crisis that adaptability gives you a decisive advantage.

Don't Become a Fossil!

Dinosaurs dominated the world 65 million years ago, until a comet 6 miles in diameter streaking 20 miles per second slammed into the Earth. The catastrophic collision instantaneously plunged the world into a very dark and cold nuclear winter that lasted for 12 months. The dinosaurs, though large and powerful, were cold-blooded and hairless, and proved incapable of adapting to the radical climate changes including a sudden and precipitous drop in temperature, and thus quickly died off in a mass extinction. In contrast, a group of small, furry, warm-blooded creatures (early mammals, and our distant ancestors) proved to be superbly adaptable to the drastic changes. Their flexibility allowed them to survive the Armageddon wrought by the comet, and when the dust finally settled, the early mammals crawled out of their burrows, squinted at the warm sun, and evolved to become the dominant creatures of the Earth. When disruptive change occurs, as it always does sooner or later in life, adaptability is often the difference between survival and extinction.

> "Life is what you make it.
> Always has been. Always will be."
> –Grandma Moses

Finding a "New Normal"

People who achieve longevity with vitality tend to know what they want and need out of life, and generally follow their own path. Typically, they are decisive, but when faced with threats and disruptive change they become flexible in their thinking, allowing them to adapt to and even embrace the changes. Kathleen, Joan's mother, was a delightful and remarkable lady who celebrated life for 99 years before leaving this realm. She was very likeable, with a good sense of humor and a graceful presence that endeared her not only to those of us in her family, but also to her friends and neighbors. Several years prior to her death, she lost her husband Leonard—the focus of her life for a half century. She reeled under the upheaval, but ultimately she found a new equilibrium, and woke up one morning several weeks later and declared, "I have found a new normal."

Kathleen's spunky and irrepressibly upbeat attitude made her a joy to be around, and she engendered affection and loyalty among almost everyone who knew her. To some degree, each of us exists in the world that we create. Her small world was full of people who made it a point to show kindness and concern for her, which gave Kathleen the strength and confidence to lead a fulfilling and independent life. She lived in and maintained her own house throughout her long life.

Bend or Break: You Decide

Hurricanes wreak havoc when they crash into coastlines, destroying most everything in their paths including massive, rigid, and sturdy oaks which are uprooted or shattered by the gale-force winds. However, the slender and pliable palm trees can bear the full force of the storm without succumbing. How can this be? A palm tree can bend over almost parallel to the ground under the force of the hurricane winds. Instead of breaking, they yield and survive to bask in the calm sunshine after the storm. In fact, scientists have discovered that these high velocity winds actually stimulate the roots of the palm tree to grow stronger and deeper.

The moral of these stories is simple: when the winds of change howl, the flexible and adaptable survive, while the stubbornly inflexible perish. Like the palm trees, Kathleen, or the early mammals, when we are faced with cataclysmic change, we need to remain adaptable and elastic so that we bend rather than break. In this way, we can not only successfully weather periods of crisis, but we can actually grow stronger and hardier in the process.

Face Your Problems

We see countless numbers of patients who, when faced with potentially devastating diagnoses such as heart disease or diabetes, rally to revolutionize their diet and lifestyle, thereby becoming much stronger and healthier than they have been in decades. The exceedingly difficult times of the 1930s forged a special group of American contemporaries. The toughness and adaptability that was demanded of them during the Great Depression helped them rise to the occasion when the world hung in the balance a few years later. This group of people, now known as the Greatest Generation, answered the call and saved the world as we know it.

Today the pace of change is dizzying for many, and our living conditions are not ideal for promoting our well-being. Almost 70 percent of American adults are overweight or obese; the health and vitality of many individuals, both grown-ups and kids, have been deteriorating as rapidly as our waistlines have been expanding. Much about this hostile change in our environment is beyond our control, but what we can and must do is remain flexible in our thinking and adjust our lives to the new realities and non-stop changes. A business-as-usual, head-in-the-sand approach is not going to help you thrive in our new and rapidly evolving world.

Americans have been unintentionally wandering down a hazardous path that led us into a place that is unfamiliar to our genetic makeup and toxic to our bodies. As a culture, we find ourselves deep in a foreboding forest, and many individuals are so bewildered they have no idea which way to turn. We have instincts, such as: move when you have to and rest whenever you can, and eat as many calories as possible every chance you get. These intuitions worked for us in the wild and natural world for which we are genetically adapted, but they will make you sick and eventually kill you in the 21st century.

Open Your Mind

In today's world you have to be open-minded enough to defy some of these counterproductive instincts and habits. Instead, try to move every chance you get, choose low-calorie, natural foods, and stop eating before you are overly full; also make your sleep a priority—try to get 7½ to 9 hours of sleep each night. These are the habits that will enable you to stay lean, strong, fit, and happy in our modern environment—there is no shortcut. Sure, it is easy to drive everywhere, ride the elevator and shun the stairs, and gulp down in 5 minutes a delicious 1,500-calorie fast-food meal for just $4. But, if you can learn to be disciplined and enlightened enough to blaze your own trail, you can live with exceptional vitality. This is a path that we need to walk down rather than drive through; one where we must slow down from time to time so we can admire the beauty of life. It is a path where we focus on investing more of our time and money on sharing enjoyable and invigorating experiences, and spend less money and energy on acquiring and maintaining material possessions.

Start with a Secure Foundation

Joan's parents, Kathleen and Leonard, were examples of the remarkable people from the Greatest Generation. Leonard, born and raised in Hawaii, didn't own a pair of shoes until he was 10. For after-school snacks, he climbed trees to pick tropical fruit and dove for abalone in the Pacific. Kathleen moved to Honolulu to work for the U.S. Navy shortly after the bombing of Pearl Harbor. After the war, Kathleen and Leonard moved to San Francisco and got married. They made a perfect pair: Leonard was a happy-go-lucky, free spirit who loved nature and worshipped his "Kitty." Kathleen, in contrast, was smart, tough-minded, and practical. When she would ask her only child, "How's it going, Joanie?" Joan would reply, "Great!" Kathleen would caution her, "Well, just wait, trouble is probably just around the corner." When her teenage daughter was being a drama queen about her dress or her hair, or whatever, Kathleen would say, "Joanie, no one is looking at you!" When Joan went away to college in San Diego, one evening she called home very distraught about a crisis in her co-ed life. Kathleen calmly listened to her and in her wise and comforting tone said, "Well, Joanie, everything is fine at home." Somehow, being reassured about the stability of the foundation of her world made her issues seem much less daunting.

Individually, we cannot remove many of our societal stresses, but we can make ourselves more stress-proof by ensuring that our foundation is secure. A nation is only as strong as the sum of her people. If we each adapt to our ever-changing world by growing healthier and more adaptable, America will grow stronger as well. Americans by nature tend to be inspired and ambitious, and we have a legacy of rallying together and rising to the occasion in times of crisis and change. The world is changing more rapidly and radically than ever before. If we adopt a resilient and optimistic outlook, we will be able to not only adjust to the new stresses but actually grow stronger because of them.

Time heals nearly everything. Sometimes when you are bogged down in the middle of an affliction, even something as minor as a cold or flu, it can seem like you might never get better, even though you have overcome many worse afflictions in the past. It is only natural to sometimes become discouraged and distressed with all of the ominous potential threats to our health and well-being today. Many people are suffering the ill effects of chronic emotional anguish, worry, and depression; and stress is now the third most common cause of heart attacks. Although the cycles of disruptive change come and go, if we can adapt to the new realities and demands, we can grow stronger because of them.

Life is like an extraordinary and sometimes frightening one-way journey on a mystery train. Nobody knows what lies ahead, and you can only count on one certainty—there is no return trip. Wrap your head around the reality that no matter how unpleasant or enjoyable your situation is today, it is bound to change soon. Particularly when you are bogged down at a station that is turning out to be difficult or unpleasant, take heart—your train will be rolling again soon, headed to an unknown station full of new possibilities. So, you are never truly stuck, even when it feels as though you might be. The train of life is in constant motion; so relax, enjoy the ride, and make the most of it. Life may not always be fair, or easy, or predictable, or even comfortable, but it is still a gift to be alive—we remind ourselves to never take that for granted. Today is our chance to blossom in the sun; embrace life and dance while you can.

> "Two wolves are fighting for your heart. One is full of anger and hatred; the other is full of love, forgiveness and peace. Which one will win? The one you feed."
> –Native American Parable

8 Ways to Shore Up Your Foundation and Safely Weather Stormy Conditions

During stressful times you will need your strength and resiliency more than ever, so take time to invest in your health and well-being. You won't be able to share the best parts of your character, talents, and personality if you don't optimally take care of yourself—body, mind, and spirit.

1. Invest in your relationships. More than any other factor, the relationships we have with the people in our lives determine our happiness and health. Eat with your family, play with your pals, call your mother, read to your kids or grandchildren (and text them too), and have lunch with your friends. Just a few relationships based on love, trust, and mutual respect can provide you with an emotional armor that will bulletproof you against

blasts of stress. Build a network of family and friends, and make it a priority to stay connected. Your job will not take care of you if you are sick or disabled, but your loved ones will. Bond with your neighbors; few things in life are as valuable as a good friend next door or just down the block. Neighborhood buddies provide a unique and mutually beneficial source of security, companionship, and friendship.

2. Forget the grudges. It doesn't take a big person to carry a grudge. A friend from Ireland said to me, "Do you know what Irish Alzheimer's is? You forget everything but the grudges." Life is too short to waste time and energy on hatred. Make peace with your past so it won't ruin the present. Forgive everyone and everything.

3. Avoid comfort/junk foods. Many people try to relieve their worries by indulging themselves with a pint of ice cream. This won't help to lower stress, it will leave you feeling guilty and physically miserable 30 minutes later. Instead, have a cup of tea, or go for a walk, or go outside and do some gardening.

4. Laugh and smile more. Sometimes, laughter is truly the best medicine. Try not to take yourself so seriously; nobody else does. A sense of humor will scare away the happiness vampires. Hearty laughter from the belly causes significant reductions in blood pressure and stress hormones like cortisol and adrenaline. You are in charge of your own happiness. Make time to do the things that you most enjoy. The activities that allow us to feel true to our nature will energize us.

5. Stay optimistic. Have faith; this too shall pass. Live in the moment. Mark Twain once wrote, "I am an old man and have known a great many devastating troubles; fortunately, most of them never actually happened." Attitudes are contagious. Try to hang around with positive and happy people, and their enthusiasm for life will rub off on you. Dan Buettner, author of

The Blue Zones, noted that among all of the healthy 100-year-olds he interviewed around the world, "There wasn't a grump in the bunch." Don't ruminate about past problems or hard times; focus on the happy ones instead.

6. <u>Be grateful, generous, and kind</u>. Karma is for real. When you send your love out into the world, it will come back to you. Slow down for a moment each day and remind yourself of the blessings in your life. The band Alabama sang, "I'm in a hurry to get things done. I rush and rush until life's no fun. All I have to do is to live and die. I'm in a hurry and don't know why." Try starting your day with a few minutes of gratitude. It will help to lower your stress level, and set a more centered and serene tone for the day.

7. <u>Get your sleep</u>. Your dreams will never come true if you don't allow yourself enough time to dream. We have always found that problems that feel dark, ominous, and disheartening after a long nerve-racking day usually seem much less daunting when we awaken fully rested and refreshed to a bright new dawn. Adequate sleep can also help keep your weight under control. One recent study involving a group of college students found that by adding 2 hours of sleep per night, they ate 300 fewer calories per day. Sleep deprivation accentuates the spikes in stress hormones like cortisol, which can cause cravings for high-calorie junk food.

8. <u>Get fit and stay active</u>. Get outside and walk. Brisk walking, for most people, is the single best exercise, one that you can and should do each day. It is an ideal activity to do with a companion, whether human or canine. And it is an exercise that you can often fit in anywhere, anytime. A walk in the morning can help you to start the day relaxed, or a mid-day stroll can dissipate work tension. After a hard day, a walk can cleanse the stress from your system, and a stroll after a meal can aid digestion. When possible, get outside daily to get some fresh air and

sunshine. You were not designed to live a mole-like existence. Outdoor activities among nature will reinvigorate you.

CHAPTER 4

Animal Friends with Benefits

A Little Thing Can Make a Very Big Difference

For the first time in 80 years my mother, Leatrice, found herself living alone after her 15-year-old dog, Gus, died. Starting about then, we noticed that she seemed to be walking less, and didn't have her usual spark. For a half a century she was the calm, gentle, and caring spirit at the center of a whirlwind of a household. But now, being by herself in her home left her feeling lonely and sometimes a little blue.

Despite our repeated pleas, Leatrice refused to consider adopting a new dog, insisting that she was too old to put up with all the inconveniences of a pet, especially the house training. So, we took matters into our own hands. With the help of our friends at the Wayside Waifs animal shelter we found Henri—a frisky, 6-pound, affectionate 3-year-old Yorkie/Poodle mix who is the cutest little dog ever. I packed him in a little carrier, boarded a plane with my sister Kerry, and a few hours later the 3 of us arrived, without any advance warning, on our my mother's doorstep. Leatrice was outraged that I had so brazenly ignored her wishes. She told us how this animal would be "a terrible inconvenience that is completely out of the question." I apologized but firmly explained that Henri's ticket was for a one-way flight; he wasn't there to visit—this was his new home.

To be sure, the first few months were a bit rocky. It took Leatrice a while to adjust to her new roomie; and sometimes we weren't sure Henri was going to win over his new best friend.

Slowly but surely, however, the tenor of our daily phone conversations changed. At first it was non-stop complaints about accidents on the rug, night-time awakenings for bathroom breaks, having to go outside walking with him, sometimes in rain, or sleet, or snow. But as time passed, she began to express how endearing it was to have Henri curl up by her feet when she snuggled into her bed at night, and how he was enthusiastically wagging his tail whenever she returned home from an errand. Or how he would give her affectionate doggy kisses when she picked him up, and how at happy hour Leatrice relaxed with a glass of wine before dinner while Henri sat on her lap and enjoyed a carrot or a little cheese.

When she discovered how much he loved to ride in the car, she brought him with her when she was out and about. Soon Henri was welcome everywhere Leatrice went—the post office, the coffee shop, the grocery store, and the homes of her friends and neighbors. Her local physician, Dr. Tony Kotnick, spontaneously remarked to me, "That little dog has been very good for your mother; I see the 2 of them out walking every day."

Now every Sunday afternoon, Leatrice and Henri visit the nursing home in her little hometown of Grafton, N.D., where the 2 of them brighten up the day for many of the residents. John, an 81-year-old man who has been unable to hear or speak since birth, may be Henri's biggest fan, as I witnessed during one of their visits recently. Henri scampered into John's room, spontaneously hopped up on the wheelchair and into his lap and excitedly licked his face. As he petted the little white dog, a tear rolled down John's cheek. He looked up and smiled at Leatrice, and in that quiet scene, in the language of the heart, an unmistakable message of joy and gratitude came through loud and clear.

Leatrice is a very social person with a nurturing soul who needs a housemate with whom she can grace with her love and attention. Henri gets her out for a walk about 4 to 6 times a day. She has become friends with other dog walkers in the neighborhood, and the local kids love to run over and pet Henri when they see the 2 of them out walking. It almost killed me when my mother would say things like, "My friends tell me that they can't believe my son would be so inconsiderate as to burden me with a new dog at my age." Although in the beginning all of us, especially Leatrice, had doubts that this little experiment would work out for the best, in fact it has exceeded our hopes. The saga of Leatrice and Henri has confirmed our convictions that pets, especially dogs or cats, can provide unique and powerful benefits for both mental and physical health. From improved fitness and weight loss, to a happier mood, better sleep, and lower blood pressure, pet ownership has been scientifically proven to be one of the best things a person can do for his or her health and sense of well-being.

For my mother, Henri was just what the doctor ordered. It is amazing how sometimes a very small thing, in this case a tiny dog named Henri, can make such a big difference in someone's life. For my patients who, like my mother, are living alone, physically inactive, and/or indoors too much of the time, I often write a prescription that reads: *"One dog. To be taken for a walk once daily (or more often as needed). Refills: unlimited. Generic substitution permitted."*

Rules for Non-Animal Lovers Who Visit Our Home and Are Irritated by Our Pets

1. This is their home, not yours.

2. If you prefer to not get hair and animal scents on your clothes, stay off the furniture.

3. We love our pets more than many people we know.

4. To you, they may be just lowly creatures, but to us, they are adopted kids who are short, furry, walk on all fours, and have difficulty speaking clearly.

5. Our 3 dogs and 3 cats are easier than our 4 kids. They don't complain about the food, never ask for money, are easier to train and tend to be more obedient, never drive our cars, don't insist on having the trendiest fashions, don't need a trillion dollars for college, and, if they get pregnant we can sell their offspring.

Why a Pet Does Your Heart Good

To one of my patients I mentioned, "Dennis, I'm glad you take your dog for a walk each day. What kind of dog is he?" Dennis replied, "He is a mix between a golden retriever and a wild night in the woods."

When we roll out of bed in the morning the first thing Joan does is go out to the kitchen to pick up and hug our little mutt Coco, who is furiously wagging her tail and giving her doggie kisses on the cheek. Then she opens the patio door and lets in our out-door cat. Joan picks up Sunny and scratches behind her ears as she strikes up a conversation, "How was the mouse hunting last night, Sun-Sun?" The orange tabby leans into Joan's neck and purrs back admiringly. Meanwhile, I'm lucky if I get a sideways glance and half-hearted "Good morning" out of Joan. I don't complain though be-cause Joan is such an animal lover, and I know all that unconditional love from the pets somehow helps to keep her hormones optimally aligned—which keeps her healthy and happy. And as the bumper sticker says, "When Momma ain't happy, ain't nobody happy."

When my son Jimmy spent a week volunteering at a local animal shelter, he talked us into adopting a pair of 4-month old Border collie puppies that have turned out to be so naughty that it's like raising convicted and unrepentant felons. That makes 3 dogs, 3 cats, and a Beta fish in the O'Keefe household. It's a lot of extra work, especially for Joan, but all the animal family members certainly add a lot of fun, energy, and love to our household. Almost nothing brightens up Joan's day better than the enthusiastic unconditional love, loyalty, and companionship of our pets. When our sons come home from their universities, the dogs greet them like best friends that they have missed desperately. While back at home with us, the boys shower our dogs and cats with love and affection—making it very clear to us how much they miss having their animal companions in their day-to-day lives.

Nurturing another living creature brings us outside of our own worries, and is a powerful source of happiness and healing. Petting a dog or cat lowers blood pressure, and can improve overall health, self-esteem, and mood. Pets seem to somehow shelter their owners from stress-related illnesses like heart disease and hypertension.

It not just the American people who are overweight, their animals are getting pudgy too. About 60 million dogs and cats in our country suffer from obesity, which increases their risks for heart disease, cancer, diabetes, and arthritis just as it does for their human companions. Studies consistently find that people who own dogs are more likely to maintain a daily exercise routine. An eager and enthusiastic exercise partner can help motivate you, indeed even obligate you, to get outdoors and do some walking or jogging even when you are really not in the mood for it. A recent study showed that dog owners who walked their dogs on a daily basis took 10 percent more steps and weighed 6 pounds less than dog owners who didn't walk their pets.

An added bonus is that dogs are a better crime deterrent than any security system in your home, and many people feel safer exercising when their dog is trotting by their side. Although pets require extra work and responsibility, most people find the unique emotional and physical benefits of adopting an animal companion to be worth the extra effort. For animal lovers, the enjoyment of owning a pet can bring a peace of mind that is not only good for your mental outlook, but great for your heart as well. Emotionally connecting with an animal friend lowers your stress hormones and increases the relaxation response. This soothes the irritated and over-reactive cardiovascular system typically seen in angry, frightened, or lonely people. Ultimately, these changes decrease the risk of heart attack, stroke, and death.

In summary, pets seem to lower your blood pressure and stress hormones, and in the long run help to protect you from heart disease, obesity, depression, and even Alzheimer's dementia. My good friend Dr. Mike Zabel, a cardiologist, e-mailed me, "I know from your previous work that pet ownership is associated with reduced stress levels and improved health. We have discussed this around the family dinner table and on occasion my 12-year-old daughter, Lauren, likes to remind us of this whenever she wants a new pet. At last count we have 12 household pets (not counting several dozen fish) including a chinchilla, a dove, a dog, and 2 guinea pigs. I wonder if there is a dose-response effect regarding pets and health?" I e-mailed Mike back saying that from personal experience if the house starts to feel like a zoo, and smell like a barn, you are likely at the point where acquiring more pets will add, rather than subtract, stress from your life.

CHAPTER 5

Your Routines
Will Determine Your Destiny

"If you do what you've always done, you'll get
what you've always gotten. It's not what we do
once in a while that shapes our lives,
but what we do consistently."
–Tony Robbins

Charles Duhigg, in his insightful book, *The Power of Habit*, tells the story of a pair of young fish who are swimming along one day, when an older fish swims by them and remarks, "Good morning; you two enjoying the water today?" The two younger fish swim along for short while before one of them looks over at the other and asks in a puzzled tone, "What the hell is water?"

Like the fish, oblivious to ever-present water in which they are immersed, each of us is unthinkingly immersed in the powerful routine of our day-to-day habits. By nature, the human brain is hard-wired to develop habits, which are analogous to the grooves and channels that are created in the earth by flowing water. Over time, the water will predictably and effortlessly flow through those ruts, which become deeper with time. Where do you want to go? Who do you want to be? Your habits will carry you to your destiny. Every day, each of us 'sleepwalks' through repeated patterns of choices and subconscious actions, yet because we take them for granted as immutable, they are invisible to us. Still, by simply looking for them, the habits become visible again. And once we can see our habits, and become aware of their consequences, it is within our power to bring them under our control.

> "We become what we do. Excellence is therefore
> more of a habit than a virtue."
> –Aristotle

The way we habitually think of ourselves, view our surroundings, and treat the people in our lives eventually creates the world in which each of us dwell. Unthinkingly, we develop habits and automatic choices that dominate our daily existence. A willingness to believe that change is possible is one of the first and essential steps towards making meaningful and lasting changes. When you believe that change is possible, and if you then begin to make the change a habit, 1 step at a time, day-by-day, change soon starts to become a reality.

Another step towards harnessing the tremendous power of habit is the realization that our habits are what we choose them to be. Once we make the decision to trade off an old and self-destructive habit for an empowering one, and begin the new habit, it increasingly becomes an automatic routine. And once that new pattern emerges, change seems not just possible, it starts to feel inevitable. Keep in mind that to develop a habit, good or bad, requires that you create a groove in your life so that the action becomes automatic, and this usually involves about 4 to 6 weeks of consistent practice. Truly, our habits are the force, which more so than anything else, carries us irresistibly towards our destiny. By harnessing the power of habits you can change almost anything—you just can't change everything, so you need to pick your battles wisely.

Cultivate healthy habits. Nothing else will so reliably create vitality, happiness, and longevity. What is it you really want or need to do: eat healthier, be more active, lose weight, trim your waistline, have a more positive and upbeat attitude, sleep deeply for 7½ to 9 hours each night, kick a tobacco habit, cut down on your drinking, die suddenly on your 100th birthday while making love to your partner? When you harness the power of habit, all of these goals are attainable (though admittedly that last one is a bit of a long-shot).

> "Forget about what you used to do.
> This is the moment you've been waiting for."
> –Jack LaLanne

The Importance of Your Routine

Vibrant good health is not a matter of luck or a gift, but grows out of your daily rituals. Over time, your habits—how you think, what you do and don't do, and what you eat and drink—are what you will become. Your life follows a trajectory and it's possible to see where you are headed decades before you arrive at your fate by examining your current habits and issues. Truly, the path that your health and well-being follow is determined more by your routines than your genes. In fact, your daily rituals will largely determine how healthy and happy you will be, how quickly you will age, what diseases you will or won't get, and how long you will live.

Up to 80 percent of what we do on a day-to-day basis is done as a matter of habit. So if you get into the right health habits you will be on a path towards a long and healthy life. But habits, good or bad, take about 4 to 6 weeks of daily repetition to develop; and, while you are in this difficult mode of trading bad habits for good ones, many people find themselves relying on will-power. But be warned: from a scientific standpoint, the problem with will-power is that its half-life is only 2 weeks, and it is soluble in alcohol; meaning that it is easy to lose your motivation and alcohol weakens your resolve.

Habits often start innocently, almost imperceptibly. Bumming a cigarette from a friend at a party, drinking a Pepsi on a hot day at the ballpark, skipping breakfast and then wolfing down a doughnut during a mid-morning break, or overeating at dinner and then spending the evening on the couch watching TV—this is how destructive habits begin. When we experience a pattern that feels pleasant and effortless, we want to repeat it. Before long this becomes the path of least effort—a groove in our daily ritual whereby an action stops being a choice and instead becomes an unconscious practice. What may have started as an innocent impulse can harden into habits so strong that they become like chains that you cannot break, sometimes even if your life depends upon it.

Health and vitality are the by-products of small endeavors, repeated consistently day in and day out. Expecting results without hard work is like trying to harvest where you have not planted. Life rewards actions and ignores excuses. The results you get will be proportional to the time and effort you invest in your nutrition and lifestyle. And, unfair as it may seem, with each passing birthday you will have to work a little harder to stay vigorous and youthful.

Reordering Your Priorities

Restoring balance in your life is essential for your health and happiness. Life in the 21st century seems to promote imbalance:

excess work and inadequate play, too many calories, not enough nourishing real food, overwhelming daily stress and not enough laughter and smiling, too much screen time and too little physical activity, too much rushing around, inadequate deep and restful sleep, too much materialism, and too little spirituality. One of the best ways to avoid getting swept away in the tide of the often self-defeating modern lifestyle is to live by the mantra: "Good Things First."

Get in the habit of prioritizing the things that will make your life better in the long run: exercise, eating breakfast each morning, nutritional food and healthy beverages, time to play, plenty of rest and relaxation, and a chance to make meaningful connections. When you make it a priority to eat and drink all the good first things first, you will find that you aren't constantly hungry. This makes it easier to resist the junk food temptations that surround you each day.

Luck Favors the Prepared

We believe that it is unlucky to be superstitious. If you want to be lucky regarding your health, invest time and energy in eating right, exercising daily, connecting positively with life around you, getting your sleep, and staying in touch with your trusted care providers. Vigorous, healthy people aren't simply lucky; they do what unhealthy people don't do. The harder you work at taking good care of yourself by making proactive lifestyle and diet practices part of your day-to-day habits, the more good luck you will have with your health as the years go by. Specific rituals can rejuvenate your life and put you on a course toward longevity with energy and verve. Believe in yourself, make a plan, and begin.

We Have Met the Enemy... and He Is Us

Prudence and Survival

As I look back over the generations of my family, a disturbing trend emerges: my female ancestors generally live well into their nineties (indeed my grandmother Dorothy O'Keefe finally succumbed only a few months shy of her 103rd birthday); but we males... well that is another story, a much shorter one. This is not a difficult pattern to recognize; these women typically were widows for anywhere from 2 to 5 decades!

> ## "I drive way too fast to worry about my cholesterol."
> —Jack (one of my less compliant patients)

Traditionally, the females in my family have coped with the inevitable stresses of life by emotionally supporting each other, focusing on their family's well-being, sipping green tea all day, having a single glass of wine before dinner, going to church on Sunday, and chanting prayers, such as the Rosary, whenever they were anxious. Meanwhile, the males were out driving too fast, smoking cigarettes, overworking, binge drinking, and diving headfirst off the second story of a houseboat into unexpectedly shallow water. Though they shared many of the same genes with their mothers, grandmothers, sisters, and aunts, the guys' behavior patterns and coping mechanisms made all the difference between remarkable longevity in the women, and tragically shortened lives in the men.

"Americans will always do the right thing—
after they have exhausted all of the alternatives."
–Winston Churchill

As one's life unfolds, prudence and moderation play a large role in determining our fate. Paradoxically, alcohol is one of the most common causes of premature death, yet it can also be a habit that helps to confer longevity and well-being. Alcohol is the proverbial double-edged sword; and no other health factor is capable of cutting so deeply in either direction depending upon how it is used. Studies that we and others have done clearly indicate that light-to-moderate alcohol consumption (ideally about 1 drink daily) is associated with lower risk of heart attack and cardiovascular death, and substantially better life expectancy. On the other hand, excessive alcohol intake or binge-drinking is toxic to one's heart and general health, and is the third leading cause of premature death among Americans, in no small part because it predisposes us to accidents of all sorts. As a teenager, after seeing how drinking devastated the lives of my grandfathers, I vowed to be very careful with alcohol. So I have always used alcohol like my parents and my Granny O'Keefe (whom I lived with for 4 years during college and medical school): just 1 glass of red wine with dinner (maybe a second glass for special occasions), and strictly avoiding driving after any alcohol ingestion.

A cautious and risk-averse attitude will likely yield significant health dividends over a lifetime. In the 3,500-year-old Greek story *The Iliad*, songs from the beautiful Sirens compelled the hero Odysseus to steer his fleet of ships into the rocky shallows where he and his men were driven asunder. Similarly, the thrill of risk-taking is a temptress that lures many of us males even today into destroying ourselves.

"A wise man sees in the misfortune
of others what he should avoid."
–Marcus Aurelius

Frequently, aging occurs in a quantum fashion, whereby a person enjoying good health suffers a catastrophic accident, and never again recovers his or her prior strength and vitality. After serving 8 years as an American President, Theodore Roosevelt, at age 54, was still a hale and hearty, remarkably vigorous man... until he ventured to the unexplored depths of the Amazon rainforest. During this ill-advised and extremely risky descent down the Brazilian 'River of Doubt,' one of America's larger-than-life leaders suffered needless injury, infection, and malnutrition all in the name of reckless adventure. Teddy survived, just barely, and when he returned home several months later, he was just a shadow of his former self. Roosevelt never fully recovered, and died prematurely just a few years later at age 60.

Sometimes I can relate to racecar driver Mario Andretti when he said, "If everything seems under control, you just aren't going fast enough." Those testosterone-fueled urges that fated many of my male ancestors have landed me in trouble too. For example, last year I racked up multiple speeding tickets (I'm embarrassed to admit how many), and one warning for running a stop sign on a bicycle. Author Tom Vanderbilt, in his book, *Traffic*, points out that we physicians as a group are the second worst drivers on the road, better only than students in our ability to avoid accidents. He speculates doctors' problems behind the wheel (despite our inflated opinions of our driving abilities) arise because we are often speeding from one emergency to another while distracted by urgent phone calls, and fatigued from sleep deprivation and long workdays.

These days I am trying to think, and drive, more like the sensible women in my family. Call me a wimp, but I no longer race my triathlon bike full-speed through the city streets, and I'm doing more walking with Joan through the neighborhood. I've quit jumping off 60-foot cliffs into the ocean, but I still love swimming in the outdoor pool as the sun comes up. Still snowboarding... but not keeping up with my daredevil sons and nephews as they fly down the mountain. And... I am definitely driving slower.

Avoid Stupid Mistakes. Be Careful and Smart

A few seconds of inattentiveness or recklessness can end or ruin your life. Be smart. Use your common sense, and try to follow these prudent habits.

1. Buckle up. Each and every time you get into an automobile.

2. Never text while driving. Avoid speaking on the phone while driving.

3. Obey the traffic laws. No speeding! I am working hard at complying with this one; not a single ticket in over a year now.

4. Be like a Boy Scout. Try to always be prepared, and follow recommended precautions.

5. Don't drink excessively. Never drink and drive.

6. Pay attention. Be cautious, attentive, and even hyper-vigilant when in the presence of potential dangers like a chainsaw, a weapon, heavy equipment, fire, or explosives.

7. Take precaution on 2 wheels. Wear a helmet, and avoid dangerously high speeds on bikes, motorcycles, etc.

8. Listen closely to your intuition. If you are feeling fear, your perceptive and prescient subconscious mind is warning you of a lurking danger.

9. See the doctor. Get a checkup with your physician each year; and make sure it includes tests of your cholesterol, blood pressure, blood sugar, and waist circumference.

10. Limit / Eliminate reckless behavior. One last lesson my daring, adventurous, life-of-the-party Uncle Jimmy taught me the hard way: Never do a swan-dive from heights in the dark into water of unknown depths.

Just Do It (Instead of Wasting Time Watching Others Do It)

Much of aging comes down to losing our abilities to perceive the beauty in our world and fully participate in its adventures, due to problems such as fading eyesight or diminished hearing, loss of balance and strength, or a vanishing ability to smell and taste. The erosion of our senses can be one of the most discouraging and frightening aspects of growing old. The directive, *"use it or lose it,"* applies not just to your muscles and brain, but also to your heart, vision, hearing, balance, and to your senses of smell and taste, even of course to your sexual function. So if you want your senses to come alive, you have to fully use them every chance you get. In a very real sense, you get what you settle for; so if you are finding it difficult to climb stairs, your body is telling you that you need to do more stair-climbing to rebuild those muscles. It is not overuse, but lack of use, that erodes our sensory capabilities, physical strength, and mental clarity as the decades go by. In other words, people don't wear out; they get rusted up from inactivity. Dust off the cobwebs by getting outside and using your phenomenal capabilities to their fullest, and you will find yourself growing stronger, sharper, and more perceptive.

Because the average American spends 4 to 6 hours daily staring blankly at a TV, one of the surest ways to stay dynamic and energetic is to get off the sofa, turn off the TV, and embrace life with all of your senses. Stay curious and active. Get outside. Taste and smell the natural goodness of fresh and real food. Get and give massages. Hug your loved ones. Watch the clouds sail overhead. Notice the scent of the fresh-cut grass and stop to smell the roses. Savor the taste of a glass of wine while you enjoy the company of a friend or loved one. Travel and seek out a variety of new experiences.

> "In the game of life, even seats on the fifty-yard line don't interest me. I came to play."
> –H. Jackson Brown

Turn Off the TV and Turn On Your Life!

Science shows that people who spend the most time watching television are the least happy in the long run. A new study looking at how our habits affect our moods came to the conclusion that happy people tend to spend more time socializing with family and friends, exercising, and reading—but tend to spend less time watching television. It's not that those who described themselves as happy didn't watch TV, but they spent much less time viewing television than did the unhappy people. Because this was just an observational study, we can't say which came first: do unhappy people watch more TV, or does too much TV make you unhappy? Still, even if we don't know for sure that turning off the TV will make you happier, it seems like a pretty savvy move if you want to lead a more interesting and active life.

Feel the Rhythm in Your Heart

I have been impressed by how people seem to derive real health benefits, both physical and mental, from incorporating music into their daily lives, whether it is in the form of dancing, singing, making, or even just listening to music. Rhythm comes naturally to us. The first sound that entered your awareness, even before you were born, was the rhythmic "lub-dub... lub-dub" of your mother's heartbeat. One hundred thousand times each day, your heart drums out the sound track of your life, most of the time only in the background of your consciousness. The average heart beats 3 billion times before it gives up the ghost; if you treat yours right, it may pump 4 billion times during a century of life.

Each of us was born with a song in our heart. You don't have to tell young kids to dance when you put on fun music, they naturally will just move to the beat. In the cold, dark winter days when our kids are getting stir crazy, we coax them down to the basement and ask them to put on upbeat music and they will dance, jump on a mini-trampoline, and Hula-Hoop themselves into a sweat without any cajoling. Rekindle that song within you; music can lift your spirits, melt stress, and lower blood pressure. Exercise can be fun when it is more like play and less like work; and dancing is all about having fun. Dancing is an ideal form of exercise. If you dance continuously for an hour you will take about 6,000 steps, which means during just 60 minutes of fun, you will have accumulated 60 percent of the recommended goal of 10,000 steps for an entire 24-hour period.

Recent research shows that regular dancing improves health on multiple levels, from improved balance and better physical fitness, to more flexibility and a brighter more energetic mood. The TV show *Dancing with the Stars* provides some dramatic examples of how dancing can improve fitness from week to week. Marie Osmond lost 31 pounds while participating in the competition. She fainted during one episode, probably because her blood pressure was getting back down to levels that her cardiovascular system had not seen since she was a teenager.

It's easier than ever to learn to dance, whether in a local dance studio or a gym, or in the comfort of your own home with the help of online options. YouTube.com is a great online resource for learning how to dance. Check out the wildly popular *The Evolution of Dance*, a wacky and entertaining video clip. Judson Laipply does a 6-minute dance medley that has been viewed 200 million times.

Listening to enjoyable and relaxing music may be a great habit for cultivating better cardiovascular health. A unique research project by Dr. Michael Miller showed that, by arousing positive emotions, joyful music has a favorable effect on the health of arteries. Mental stress causes the blood vessels to constrict and thereby reducing blood flow to vital organs. In this study, volunteers listened to 30 minutes of music they had previously chosen as fun and pleasant. The improvement in arterial blood flow with enjoyable music was about the same as that noted with 30 minutes of aerobic exercise or taking statin (cholesterol-lowering) medications, and greater than the benefits noted with meditation. Music, like laughter, can evoke positive feelings that offset the negative stresses of everyday life. A perfect way to double your heart health benefits is to exercise while you are listening to uplifting and energizing music.

Everyone in our family loves music; we find that just listening to music and/or singing along to songs that we enjoy makes us relaxed and happy. We don't dance in public as much as we would like to, and Joan jokes that I am choreographically challenged. A lot of people are self-conscious about getting up and dancing in front of a crowd. Even Chris Martin, the lead singer for the band Coldplay, when asked about his dancing onstage at their concerts said, "I'd get sent home from the first audition of *So You Think You Can Dance?* My dancing is sort of controlled spasms. I fully accept that it might appear ridiculous. But it's passionate."

A patient once complained during an office visit that he was too shy to square dance. His wife looked over at him and said, "Orville, get over it; nobody's watching you! So just relax and have fun." Think of dancing as a chance for physical play. Dancing is like smiling and laughing, even if you are in a bad mood, if you force yourself to do it, it won't be long before you begin to feel happier. Fitness, balance, rhythm, romance, and fun—dancing can do it all for us, we just have to get over our inhibitions and let the music move our bodies. One of our goals in life is to someday learn how to dance well.

Sitting Is the New Smoking: It's Time to Kick This Habit, Too!

I have always had a difficult time sitting still for more than a few minutes. Slouching in a chair in front of a computer and keyboard, or sitting and staring at a TV screen for more than 20 minutes makes me feel miserable. Maybe that qualifies me as hyperactive, but seated inactivity just feels uncomfortable to me.

Startling new research shows that sitting for prolonged periods of time is hazardous to your health, even if you make a point of getting in a daily workout. The adverse health effects of physical inactivity occur quickly and are severe. The metabolic activity of the body slows, your sensitivity to insulin becomes impaired and dangerous free radicals begin to rise in your bloodstream within hours of physical inactivity. In essence, too much sitting results in inflammation throughout your system, and eventually increases risks of obesity, depression, diabetes, high blood pressure, cardiac disease, and Alzheimer's dementia.

An 8-year study that followed a quarter-million American adults correlated daily activity levels with long-term general health. One of the best predictors of survival and overall health was the amount of physical activity participants did on a daily basis. Television viewing time is a great marker for sedentary behavior. The study participants who watched TV at least 7 hours per day had markedly higher risks for early death, disease, and disability compared to those who watched less television.

Prolonged sitting causes problems for almost anyone, including people who exercise regularly. Even those who exercised for 7 hours or more a week but spent at least 7 hours a day in front of the television were more likely to die prematurely than people who exercised at least 7 hours weekly and watched less than an hour of television daily.

A large study of Australians showed every hour of TV viewing can be expected to shorten a person's life by about 22 minutes. This means that if the average adult person watched no TV, he or she would probably live about 1.5 to 2 years longer. And this doesn't even take into account the fact that all those extra hours freed up might be spent in activities that bring meaning and vitality to life, such as time spent cultivating relationships with family and friends, pursuing hobbies, being active outdoors, traveling, etc.

Other research shows that simply getting off one's duff to stand or stroll for a couple of minutes every 20 minutes—no significant exertion required—will help to keep blood sugars and blood pressure lower during the day. Indeed, even just standing rather than sitting while you work will burn hundreds of extra calories over the course of a single day.

It is becoming increasingly clear that we would all be better off if we make it a point to get out of our chairs more often during the day. Steve Jobs, one of the real creative geniuses of our age, made it a point to routinely invite his colleagues and coworkers to go outside for strolls around the campus of Apple's headquarters while conducting business discussions or meetings. When on conference calls, I will often step outside and saunter through the gardens surrounding our medical center, or climb the office stairs while having phone discussions. Gretchen Reynolds, a fitness writer for the *New York Times*, works and studies while standing, by placing her reading materials on a wire music stand; she also brushes her teeth while standing on one foot to improve her balance.

So throughout the day, make it a point to move frequently, even if only to stand up for a few minutes at a time. This will help to maintain normal and steady glucose and insulin levels, and keep the nasty fats out of your bloodstream, as well as off your belly. It will also boost your mood and help to ensure your mind stays sharp. More movement, less time spent sitting, and fewer hours watching TV (no more than 2 hours a day); then, start making plans for the extra years of exhilarating life you will be earning for your efforts.

CHAPTER 6

The Best of Both Worlds

This chapter will describe how to thrive and achieve longevity with vitality by emulating the diet and lifestyle of your ancient hunter-gatherer ancestors in addition to tapping into the wonders of modern science.

How to Doctor Yourself

My great grandfather, Henry O'Keefe, was a pioneer doctor in rural North Dakota. When he went out on a house call in the winter, he usually did so in a horse-drawn sleigh. One of Henry's sons, Emmet (my grandfather), also became a doctor, and shortly after finishing his training, he nearly died from tuberculosis (TB), a disease he contracted from one of his patients. One hundred years ago, the average American didn't make it past age 47, and the 3 leading causes of death were all bacterial infections: pneumonia, tuberculosis, and dysentery (infectious diarrhea). Although today's antibiotics can almost always cure these infections, none of these drugs existed only 2 to 3 generations ago when my grandfathers were practicing medicine. Back then, physicians tended to have shorter lives than the general population owing to the fact that many of the patients they saw on a daily basis had contagious, potentially life-threatening infectious diseases for which no effective treatments existed—talk about occupational hazards!

In contrast, doctors in the U.S. today are fitter, leaner, and can expect to live longer than the average American. Indeed, in a recent study of 4 million American males, physicians had a longer life expectancy than any other occupation. When my colleagues and I did our own study on what might explain this surprising finding, we discovered that only 1 to 2 percent of American doctors smoke tobacco, compared to 23 percent of the general population. Also, American physicians tend to be sticklers about keeping their own blood pressures and cholesterol levels in the ideal ranges, and we have no reservations whatsoever about taking prescription medications to do so. We tend to stay up to date on our vaccinations, eat healthier, and exercise more than the average Joe or Jane, and thus we have lower rates of obesity and diabetes.

Not that we physicians don't have issues of our own. We tend to work long hours and often are faced with stressful situations on a daily basis. And, we often ignore the advice that says, "A doctor who treats himself has a fool for a patient." Dr. Edward Creagan from the Mayo Clinic says, "As a profession, we have not always taken good care of ourselves." Through the decades, we doctors have sometimes had to learn the hard way that we must invest the time and energy needed to stay emotionally and physically strong. Dr. Creagan points out that there is a growing awareness among physicians that, "If one is not psychologically, spiritually, and physically fit, one will not go the distance in this profession."

I was explaining the increased longevity of modern-day physicians to a group of doctors at a medical meeting recently when one of them quipped, "I sacrificed my young adulthood buried in medical textbooks and staying up all night taking call in hospitals. It's gratifying to know that I may get some of that time back at the other end of my life." A different physician in the audience chimed in to say, "I'm not sure that missing out on our 20s in exchange for an extra decade in our 80s is such a great trade!" The crowd of doctors roared with laughter.

Medicine has made mind-boggling progress when one considers how far and how fast we have come in just the past few decades. No aspect of medicine has made more progress than preventive care, although its power and effectiveness are often overlooked and generally underappreciated, in part because American medicine rewards care providers much more generously for treating acute illnesses than for preventing the health catastrophes in the first place. However, we doctors see firsthand how important, effective, and indispensable a prudent diet, regular exercise, and modern therapies to control risk factors are to health and well-being; and so we are increasingly applying these preventive measures to our own lives.

Living in 21st century America reminds me of the opening line from Charles Dickens' *A Tale of Two Cities*, "It was the best of times, it was the worst of times." Obesity, diabetes, depression, high blood pressure, and Alzheimer's disease are more common than ever before and the rates of these epidemics are still rising. Yet if one pays close attention, each of us has a better chance of living a longer, more active, and enjoyable life than at any time in the 150,000 years that our species, *Homo sapiens*, has walked the planet Earth. The key is following the path less traveled—one that involves embracing the modern technologies to overcome any health issues that might arise, all the while imitating the diet and exercise patterns of our ancient ancestors who lived in the wild.

Life can be hard, but it will surely get harder if you are careless with your health. On the other hand, if you are smart about taking care of yourself, your life is likely to be long and healthy. In reality, what we are all interested in is not so much lifespan as health-span—the number of high-quality years of life we get to enjoy. Don't believe the old adage: live fast, die young, and save yourself from a decade in diapers strapped into a wheelchair in the nursing home. It turns out that the best way to live a full, dynamic, active, and fully-functional life is the same strategy for living to a ripe old age. If you do the right things this morning, you will start to feel better by this afternoon; you won't have to wait until you are 80 to realize the benefits.

Fear Is Darkness, Knowledge Is Light

Uncertainty, particularly where it concerns your health or that of a loved one, often leads to fear and anxiety. Fear can disable you, and diminish the joy and confidence you need to fully enjoy and participate in life. Harness the power of knowledge, and you will have the courage to live boldly. When you are frightened about your health, you need to seek answers rooted in powerful 21st century science. Knowledge can banish fear and increase your chances of living with the warm glow of great health. Knowledge can also channel any anxiety you have into motivation to do what you need to do in order to not just survive but to thrive with vigor and longevity.

When I was in college and medical school, I subconsciously tried to pretend that I didn't have any issues, hoping that if I ignored my high cholesterol or high-normal blood pressure, the problems might just magically disappear. Men in particular seem predisposed to this *if it ain't broke, don't fix it* approach to their health, though we instinctively understand the necessity and power of preventive maintenance for the house or car.

"Life is a journey not a destination;
and the road is always under construction."
–Keith Cameron Smith

Honestly, I am not sure how well the *'head in the sand'* approach works for the ostrich, but it usually turns out to be a disastrous strategy for human health. Fortunately, after practicing medicine for just a few years I realized that everyone has his or her own health issues. Some people choose to ignore them, and sooner or later, that approach usually doesn't end well. I recall having a bedside discussion with a man who had recently suffered a heart attack, his wife looked over at him and said, "When it comes to his notions about health, my husband reminds me of a stopped clock—occasionally right, but mostly wrong." Instead you should strive to discover and address your particular issues, often with the help of one or more trusted professional advisors. The *'knowledge is power'* strategy puts you on a trajectory for an enjoyable, fully self-actualized, and lengthy journey through life. Although we will all experience some unavoidable and unexpected turbulence from time to time, 75 percent or more of chronic health issues can be brought under control and neutralized. Still, many people make the mistake of choosing the path of least effort, and thus don't make it a priority to follow a good diet and exercise and fail to objectively assess and follow their important health and fitness metrics like blood pressure, cholesterol, blood sugar, and waist circumference.

In Italy during the Middle Ages, a profession known as a *codega* existed. People would hire a *codega* for security and protection to walk in front of them with a lantern to show the way, and frighten away thieves and other dangers that might be lurking in the dark shadows of the night. Think of your doctor, trainer, or dietitian as a modern day *codega*. We are here to light your way and make sure your joy of life and future well-being are not ambushed by some silent stalker like cancer, heart attack, stroke, high blood pressure, high cholesterol, or diabetes. These and other health issues can only darken your future if you passively allow them to do so by ignoring them today.

"He who conceals his disease
cannot expect to be cured."
–Ethiopian Proverb

While you are striving to become the best you can be, don't ignore the single best source of objective information about your health—your medical checkups. Think of your medical visits in a positive light—you need this kind of feedback to be the best you can be. We can help you to grow into a healthier person, a better athlete, a more valuable employee, a more dynamic parent or grandparent, a more resilient traveler, a more passionate lover, or whatever it is that you would like to become. Take responsibility for your wellness. Be vigilant and proactive about finding high-quality medical care and get regular feedback about your health numbers and issues. Discovering and addressing any potential risks and/or chronic health conditions you might have are essential for ensuring your bright and healthy future.

As doctors, we can reassure you with our assessments, but peace of mind and self-confidence about your wellness and resilience are feelings that you create within yourself. True confidence in your health and physical capabilities is something you earn by setting moderately difficult personal goals and incorporating a variety of exercise and healthy foods and beverages into your daily routine. Self-assurance comes from proving yourself to you. Life is short, and today is meant to be your moment in the sun. The feeling of strength and vitality coursing through your body engenders a sense of security and confidence in your ability to handle whatever life demands of you. And this kind of confidence will also allow you to enjoy life to its fullest.

Are Your Numbers Ideal?

The 21st century is the Digital Age, and numbers dominate our existence—cell phones, credit cards, door codes, dates and times, interest rates, taxes, bank accounts, social security, and your weight. Yet, the most crucial numbers of your life often remain out of sight and out of mind. The numbers that will determine your long-term health and longevity are blood pressure, cholesterol, triglycerides, glucose, and waist size. If you can keep these critically important health numbers in their ideal ranges your well-being and life expectancy will be dramatically improved. Face it, your health and well-being are more important to you than to anyone else; so if you want optimal health it's an issue in which you must take ownership. And don't assume you can ignore these numbers until they start to bother you—by then it's often too late. This is why it is so important that you proactively track these levels, and make sure that your crucial numbers are in the ranges that lead to vigor and longevity. These key vital signs will determine whether your brain, heart, kidneys, blood vessels, and liver will stay strong and youthful through the decades:

Ideal Ranges

Total Cholesterol	LDL Cholesterol	Systolic Blood Pressure (top number)	Fasting Blood Sugar (after 12 hours of not eating)	Waist Circumference (Measure waist size 1 to 2 inches above belly button)
Less than 180	40 to 100	95 to 130	Less than 100	Less than half of height in inches divided by 2*

* If you are 5 feet 8 inches your waist circumference should be less than 34 inches.

If you need help in shifting these important numbers into ideal ranges (and most people do), Becky Captain, APP, and our staff in the Duboc Cardio Wellness Clinic at Saint Luke's Hospital in Kansas City are eager to see that you achieve your goals using safe, easy to tolerate, and proven strategies. Becky is among the most knowledgeable and effective experts in cardiac prevention in America, and the patients that she sees on a regular basis virtually always stay healthy and avoid chronic illness and disability. The American health care system is really designed to be more of a disease care system—set up to address and treat acute problems. So if you want to thrive, not just survive, in the long run you will need to take it upon yourself to develop healthy habits. If you can follow all 4 of the essential lifestyle recommendations you will be in the top 3 percent of Americans. These recommendations are: 1) not smoking, 2) maintaining a healthy weight, 3) eating at least 5 servings of vegetables and fruits each day, and 4) exercising at least 30 minutes daily. If, instead, you come up with excuses why you can't make these 4 fundamentals a reality, you may end up in the same boat as the other 97 percent of people who are suffering from rising rates of obesity, diabetes, heart disease, and other chronic illnesses.

Optimize your health numbers with the help of a trusted prevention-oriented physician. Do your best with diet and exercise, but when deemed necessary, don't hesitate to take one or more safe and effective prescription medications that might be needed to get these numbers in their ideal ranges. The availability of powerful and well-tolerated drugs to normalize these risk factors is the most important reason that we are living longer and healthier lives than ever before. Do not deprive yourself of this major advantage of living in the 21st century. Most of the healthiest middle-aged and older people I know are taking one or more of these medicines that will allow them to stay fully functional and alive for decades to come. Get regular check-ups and do the recommended screening procedures like mammograms, colonoscopies, PAP smears, bone density testing, CardioScan (coronary calcium score), and routine blood work.

It's Your Blood Pressure, Get to Know It!

Nine out of 10 Americans develop high blood pressure sooner or later, so it is crucial that you keep track of this easily obtainable vital sign. The most important blood pressure reading is not the one done in your doctor's office, or your local drug store, but rather your average blood pressure throughout your day-to-day life. In that regard, ideally you should keep a blood pressure monitor in your house and keep track of your blood pressure from time to time.

If you have high blood pressure and are having difficulties controlling it, you may need to check it more than once a day. It's very useful to keep a log of your blood pressures, and bring this into your doctor when you show up for your follow-up visits. I find it extremely helpful to have my patients bring in an extensive log of their blood pressures obtained at different times and places over several weeks. Don't check your blood pressure only when you are feeling relaxed and happy, but also at times when you're feeling stressed, sleep deprived, angry, tired, and anxious. A list of blood pressures is invaluable when your physician and you are deciding whether or not your blood pressure control is adequate.

One of the best manufacturers of home monitors is Omron®; these are reliable machines that automatically inflate and deflate and record precise and reproducible measurements of blood pressure and heart rate. I would suggest that you purchase one of their less expensive models (3 Series or 5 Series). The higher end models have more bells and whistles, but these are generally unnecessary. Use only an upper arm cuff; the wrist cuffs are less accurate.

When taking your blood pressure, you should be seated and relaxed with your arm resting comfortably on a table at approximately the level of your heart (or your left breast). Both feet should be flat on the floor. Check your blood pressure 2 to 3 times, about a minute or 2 apart. Generally, we recommend that you throw out the first reading. An average of the subsequent 2 or 3 readings is the most accurate estimate of your blood pressure. Ideal blood pressure is 100 to 130 for the top number and 55 to 85 for the bottom number. Occasionally, your readings will be outside this ideal range, and that's okay—blood pressure is highly variable depending on what you are doing and how you are feeling at the moment, so it will sometimes be higher and at other times lower. The important thing is that most of your blood pressure readings are in the ideal range. We can nearly always achieve this by working with you on your diet and lifestyle and sometimes using one or more medications as necessary. Your blood pressure is perhaps your most important vital sign, so don't take it for granted. Keeping your blood pressure in the ideal range is one of the most important things you can do to safeguard your long-term health.

CHAPTER 7

Strength from Nature:
May the Force Be with You

This year our family vacationed on a Caribbean island, where I spent at least an hour each day swimming and snorkeling in the crystal clear waters off the pristine white sand beaches. I love swimming in the ocean, especially when the water is clear enough to see the amazing underwater world teeming with diverse marine life. Part of the exhilaration I feel while swimming in the deep blue sea comes from an adrenaline rush induced by the realization that this is virtually the only time and place that I, as a modern human being, am immersed back in the natural food chain—and not at the top! And that survival-of-the-fittest state of mind sharpens my senses, keeps me focused on the moment, and makes me feel acutely alive.

For the first time in the history of humankind, most of the people on the planet live in urban rather than rural settings, where crowding and a 24/7 nonstop, frenetic pace in a man-made world typically lead to stress and anxiety. Richard Louv, author of the book *The Nature Principle*, says, "Time spent in nature is one of the only real, consistent, inexpensive antidotes to the burnout we are feeling." A growing body of evidence suggests that getting outdoors in Earth's native environments can be a healing therapy that can improve both physical and mental health. In fact, a new field of medicine, dubbed *eco-therapy* or nature therapy, indicates that Mother Nature may turn out to be among the most powerful sources of healing and renewal. Time spent being physically active outdoors helps to lift depression, alleviates anxiety, reduces stress, and lowers blood pressure. In fact, if you want to improve your overall health and well-being, it is hard to beat getting out in nature, even if only for short periods of time, like 10 to 15 minutes, at least once during each day.

The Force Runs Strong in You

The Force, as depicted in the classic *Star Wars* movie series, is an energy field created by living beings that surrounds us and binds all life together. According to this legend, for those who learn to channel its power, the Force can enhance our natural physical and mental abilities, like strength and wisdom. Since the first time I saw that ground-breaking movie in 1977, I have been charmed by the idea that we can learn to feel the Force all around us. Yoda, while teaching the young Luke Skywalker to train his body as well as his mind, tells Luke, "a Jedi warrior's strength flows from the Force." Today we spend far too much time sitting in front of screens or behind windshields, which in *Star Wars*' lingo, has caused "a great disturbance in the Force." Modern technology and indoor sedentary lifestyles isolate us from our natural world. Strength, tranquility, serenity, wisdom, inspiration, healing, and vigor can flow from the force that emanates from all living organisms. I personally can feel the benefits of connecting with other living beings, including plants and animals, and I also see their positive effects among my family, friends, and patients.

My mother, Leatrice, and her beloved dog companion, Henri, go outside for a walk 4 or 5 times a day, even when it means venturing out into the snowy and frigid cold North Dakota winter nights—something she would, at age 83, never even think of doing on her own. My patient and friend, George, is an avid gardener who finds that tending plants brings him a sense of purpose and contentment like nothing else does. Over the 20 years during which I have cared for him, he has survived 2 cancers, a heart attack, open-heart surgery, and a major vascular surgery. Though he has always lived alone, each day he nurtures his gardens and houseplants with devotion and love. Also, nearly every day George eats fresh and/or canned vegetables and fruits that he has grown and harvested himself. I believe it is the physical and emotional strength that he draws from his connectedness to his plants that has allowed him to repeatedly overcome long odds and triumph over threats to his life like lung cancer, lymphoma, heart disease, and an aortic aneurysm.

Immersion in nature awakens our senses and resonates profoundly with something deep within our being. This stimulates creativity and intelligence, and energizes and rejuvenates us. Our natural world is filled with mysterious natural phenomena and marvelous life forms, all of which we are connected to through an intricate web of life on Earth. Feel the wind moving over the land, and hear the soft rustling of the leaves in the trees. Enjoy the sensation of your skin soaking up warm sunshine, or the coolness of soft mist falling on your face. The patterns and connectedness of the natural world makes us realize that we belong here; that we are part of something much larger than each of us.

Being active outdoors in nature enlivens and relaxes us at the same time. The wonderment of looking across a lake or out at an ocean can make our everyday anxieties seem much less daunting. Natural spaces are inherently less stressful because they provide native and rhythmic stimuli, such as the sounds of waves rolling onto a shoreline, a babbling brook, or birds singing over-head and crickets chirping on the ground, or the sight of billow-ing clouds sailing peacefully across the sky. These sensations bring deep relaxation, calming the racing thoughts provoked by the overstimulation of our modern world. This can free up space for you to breathe deeply and think more clearly.

Sometimes, I will wear my iPod when I am out running or walking, but I have learned that outdoor exercise, especially when I am out in a natural setting, leaves me much more relaxed and invigorated when I listen to the sounds of nature. There is some-thing magical about just taking in the sky, the clouds, the sun, the fresh air, and the trees.

Go Outside and Play

Even if you are not up for epic adventures into the wilderness, make a habit of taking at least a few minutes to get outside for some nature therapy at least once or twice daily. If you think you don't like the outdoors I'd suggest that maybe you haven't found your right way of experiencing it, or the right place. There is virtually no weather that keeps me indoors; it's just a matter of dressing appropriately. And here in the middle of the USA, we get a wide variety of weather during 4 distinctly different seasons, which I find imbues life with a reassuring natural cyclical rhythm. Taking a brisk walk in a nearby park, or just along a tree-lined street can provide benefits, both immediate and long-term, to your health and happiness. Getting outside in any natural environment can be restorative, even if it is nothing more than small green space in the middle of an otherwise drab, bustling urban asphalt and concrete metropolis. The key is to move your body once you find a natural sanctuary. Green exercise—walking, running, biking, swimming, gardening, stretching, etc., in an outdoor natural setting, will boost your mood and self-esteem, and, over time, can dramatically improve your physical and mental health and well-being. Get outdoors among nature every day. Here are a few suggestions:

1. Sometimes walk or bike to your destination; try to make part of the trip through an area that has trees and grass along your route.

2. Visit a nearby park, or any green space, during breaks in your workday, for example: over the lunch hour, during coffee, or immediately after finishing work.

3. Plant a garden and nurture plants in your yard and inside your home. If you live in an apartment, check out books on container gardening for small spaces.

4. Take vacations to naturally beautiful locations.

5. Take your dog outside for walks regularly.

6. Eat outside whenever you get the chance.

7. Sit or work by a window with a view of a natural setting whenever you get the opportunity.

8. Instead of always meeting indoors, occasionally go for an outdoor walk with a colleague or co-worker while you discuss an issue.

9. Make a point of appreciating or commenting on natural splendor such as a gorgeous sunset, a majestic oak, a beautiful garden, or a brilliant moon.

Natural Cycles Bring Your Life Back into Balance

This planet paradise is our one true home and its natural cycles have been intertwined with ours throughout humanity's existence—that is until very recently. Many Americans today have fallen out of step with the natural cycles of our world, leaving them emotionally and physically unwell.

In nature, everything is circular and connected. Our perfectly spherical Earth spins around on its axis every 24 hours, and circles the sun every 365 days. Water circulates down from the clouds, bringing life to the land and then evaporates back into the sky, being purified in its cycle. In the intricately connected, awe-inspiring cycle of life, plants grow and prosper by using water and sunshine combined with 2 animal waste products—nitrogen and carbon dioxide; and the plants reciprocate by giving off oxygen and bearing the vegetables, fruits, seeds, and nuts that we animals need to thrive. Early native human cultures instinctively understood that they were part of these cyclical, interconnected rhythms, living in their round shelters, dancing in circles around the campfire ring, going about their daily rounds while hunting and gathering.

Indigenous cultures in ages past and even today are still more connected and respectful of nature this way.

In contrast, our modern, man-made environments have
detached many of these vital connections to our natural circular,
cyclical world. Today our lives are defined by boxes, not circles. If
you are like most Americans, you probably awaken in the box that
is your bedroom and get your breakfast from a box. You climb
into a box on wheels and go to a larger box, where you work in a
cubicle, staring at a computer box for much of the day. Then you
come back to your box of a home and stare at another box for
entertainment. It is time to break out of the box and reconnect with
the cycles of nature.

Love Life, and It Will Love You Back

Winter is the season most dominated by the boxy indoor
existence, but this gives way to spring when our native environment explodes into green and the birdsongs announce that life is
being reborn anew. Celebrate your place in this miraculous world
by getting outside. Let the warm sunshine and fresh air rejuvenate
you. Walk, run, or cycle around the neighborhood or a nearby park.
Beginning in March, for people living north of the line of latitude
from Atlanta to Los Angeles, the sun climbs high enough in the sky
to stimulate the production of Vitamin D in your skin again. When
the sun is high in the sky it only takes 15 to 30 minutes of sun at
least a few times a week to boost your level of this key nutrient,
which is vitally important for the health of everything from your
bones and your immunity to your heart.

Plant a garden or a fruit tree. Food that you grow yourself
invigorates your health long before it ever makes it to your plate.
The physical benefits of digging in the earth and the unique sense of
happiness that comes from nurturing other life are benefits you can't
get from a pill. Eat fresh plants like fruits, berries, nuts, and vegetables, especially the leafy green ones. Visit the farmer's market where

you will find fresh whole foods, not processed modern fare made from food harvested long ago and far away. Drink pure water and feel its goodness circulate through you and cleanse your system.

Consider sharing your wisdom and mentoring a younger person. Connecting with people from generations older and younger than yours will broaden your perspectives and strengthen ties. Don't let your heart run out of summers; revitalize your existence and reach your full potential by re-synching your biorhythms with the natural cycles of life.

Nurturing Nature: Good for Your Heart and Soul

Spring has always been my favorite season. The tall-grass plains of northeastern North Dakota where I grew up become harsh, frozen tundra during the winter. When spring would finally arrive my mother, Leatrice, would send me and my siblings outside saying, "This glorious spring weather just makes you happy to be alive!" Spring is the time to awaken from hibernation, shake off our dreary, sluggish attitudes and renew our enthusiasm for life. It's the season for growth and rejuvenation when the earth grows young again and we can too. Get outside among the new, bright green foliage and lovely blossoms, listen to the birds singing in trees, feel the sunshine warm upon your skin, and breathe deeply the fresh clean air. Don't be misled by the dermatology world, which teaches that sunshine is evil and toxic; we were designed by nature to be outside in the sun. Reconnecting with nature in springtime is not only good for curing your winter blues, it's a great way to grow physically stronger as well.

Recently, we were at a dinner party and the topic of gardening came up. It was fun to see our friend Rick's eyes light up as he told us about his rose gardens. In springtime he is out there working the soil, preparing the beds, watering, fertilizing, and trimming the rosebushes. It is one of his passions in life and he insists that it is a spiritual experience—good for his soul, as he puts it.

Nurturing other life, whether it be tending plants, playing with your children or grandchildren, or taking your dog for a walk, does your heart good. And it is not just the physical exercise that confers the benefits. Caring for life around you and watching it thrive and bloom in response to your kindness, compassion, and love can be one of the real joys in life. This kind of exercise has the power to change your hormonal profile, lowering the stress hormones and amplifying the hormones that promote relaxation and strengthen your immune system. Also, gardening is a great way you can give back to Mother Earth. Photosynthesis, the process that produces the energy to power plant life, consumes carbon dioxide and produces oxygen as a waste byproduct. Thus, by planting and growing trees, gardens, and lawns we are increasing the oxygen in our atmosphere and helping to protect Earth from global warming.

The number 1 leisure time physical activity in the U.S. is gardening. This is great news because gardening may be one of the very best things you can do to improve your overall well-being. While you're mowing the lawn, trimming trees and bushes, planting flowers in pots, pulling weeds, raking leaves, digging soil, watering, spreading fertilizer, or just appreciating the fruits of your labor in the form of beautiful foliage and delicious produce, gardening has the power to make you thrive and grow healthy again, just like the plants you are nurturing.

Gardening involves light-to-moderate and sometimes even strenuous exercise that incorporates many important elements of an ideal fitness program such as stretching, balance, aerobic conditioning, and strength training. Regular garden chores can burn anywhere from 200 to 400 calories each hour depending on the intensity of the activity. Gardening is nature's version of cross-training: but it demands that we lift bags of dirt instead of iron dumbbells, that we walk behind a mower instead of on a treadmill, and that we stretch to trim those higher and lower branches instead of doing yoga. A recent survey of 2,000 British people reported that 84 percent of them felt instantly relaxed when they were out in nature. When we are out working or playing in natural outdoor surroundings we tend to be happier and more relaxed. When I was a teenager, I spent every summer working at a local greenhouse/nursery, planting and caring for trees, bushes, and flowers throughout the small town in which I grew up. It instilled in me a love of plants, and now more than ever, I find that nurturing my quiet green friends brings me peace and contentment.

An Upside to Tough Times

If you are cringing as you pump gasoline at $4 a gallon into your car's fuel tank, you might take solace in the fact that scarcity sometimes can be a blessing in disguise. Heart disease deaths skyrocketed for much of the 20th century, except for the lean years that began with the Great Depression and ended after World War II. Curiously, Americans' hearts grew stronger and healthier during those trying times between 1929 and 1945—and certainly not because of lower stress levels.

Scientists studying this unexpected reprieve from the epidemic of heart disease came to the conclusion that it was the rationing of sugar, butter, meat, and gasoline that halted the march of coronary artery disease across the land. During that harsh economic era, Americans typically ate less of most foods, especially meat and processed carbohydrates, but did eat more locally caught fish and home-grown vegetables. And because gasoline was limited, they restricted their driving habits, and used their bodies for locomotion.

I recall my grandmother's stories about life in the 1930s and 40s and how she relied on carrots, tomatoes, asparagus, potatoes, beans, and beets from her garden to help feed her family. A staple in her diet was lettuce soup, which she often made for me while I was living with her while attending medical school. For many years Dorothy, who lived to be 103, also walked to and from her workplace each day (2.5 miles round trip), because her legs were the only transportation option she could afford.

If we can respond to some harsh economic realities as they come and go with the same frugal and industrious spirit as our ancestors, we will reap the health benefits as they did. Do less driving and more walking. Try to walk for some local errands, or ride a bike to the store when you need just a few items. Plant a garden, play in the dirt, and bask in the sun.

The Hygienic Theory

Headlines warn us on a daily basis of potential killer SARS or bird flu pandemics looming on the horizon or MRSA Staph Aurous bacteria that are evolving resistances to all known antibiotics. So it's not surprising that antibiotic soaps, antiseptic wipes, hygienic face masks, disposable gloves, and high-tech indoor air filters are all the rage with germophobic Americans. However, some of the most common ailments today may be due to the fact that we don't get enough exposure to the friendly germs out in the natural world. The hygiene theory postulates that, the rise in asthma, allergies, and other autoimmune diseases is in part due to the fact that by living in our sterile man-made, indoor urban dwellings, we are increasingly more isolated from nature. Our immune system is designed to be constantly interacting with a wide variety of antigens from the natural environment, like those found in soil and on animals and plants. These days we obsess about trying to make our world more antiseptic and sterile when in fact our body thrives on just the opposite—the friendly bacteria and antigens found in nature on the plants, animals, and soil.

To be clear, we're not talking about hanging out on overcrowded germ-ridden jet airliners or drinking contaminated water. But this is just one more reason to embrace gardening and other outdoor activities, and adopt animals to live with you in your house. The hard work required to digest fresh whole natural plants is exactly what is needed to keep your gut healthy. Paradoxically, a diet of easily digested processed foods like sugar and white flour, predisposes to problems like constipation, ulcers, diverticulosis, and cancer. When you spare your musculoskeletal system the stress and pounding of hard physical work like lifting, running, bending, and stretching it doesn't grow healthier; it atrophies and becomes weak and diseased. So too, your immune system needs exercise to stay strong and capable. The healthiest way to keep your immune system tuned up is to get outside and immerse yourself in the natural environment.

Prebiotics and Probiotics

Your body is made up of about 10 trillion cells working together in an incomprehensively complex and intelligently choreographed collaboration. Still more astounding is the fact that hiding in the nooks and crannies of our body (particularly in the bowels) we have at least 100 trillion foreign, non-self, cells within us or attached to us. These bugs are neither dangerous parasites nor passive passengers but rather important collaborators in our struggle for health and survival. These healthy bacteria work together with our own cells in a symbiotic relationship that keeps disease at bay and helps us to digest food and nourish us. A study in the February 24, 2011, issue of the *New England Journal of Medicine* reported that children who grew up in the country and were exposed to more soil and a variety of microbes in their everyday environment had 50 to 75 percent lower rates of asthma and allergies as adults compared to city kids who didn't get exposed to dirt and nature. The hygiene theory has also been called the *eat dirt hypothesis*, which reasons that natural germs help to strengthen the immune system and thus offer protection against autoimmune diseases as well as asthma and allergies.

Many bacteria, for instance lactobacillus and bifido-bacterium, are friendly microbes that set up camp in our gut and help us to digest food, prevent dangerous infections, and appear to benefit even the health of our lungs, blood pressure, heart, and reproductive organs. These normal healthy gut bacteria are called *probiotics*. They have long been known to promote digestive health and to support a strong and vigilant immune system. Some recent research suggests that probiotics can also help to lower cholesterol and blood pressure, and prevent lung infections.

Prebiotics is a term used for natural, healthy plant fibers that would be indigestible without the help of healthy gut bacteria. These fibers help to provide an ideal environment in which the healthy bacteria can thrive. The combination of prebiotics (soluble fiber) and probiotics (healthy bacteria) in your daily diet can bring about several health benefits including: fewer symptoms of irritable bowel syndrome (such as cramping, diarrhea, and constipation), lower risks for stomach ulcers and ulcerative colitis, reduced number and severity of urinary and lung infections, lower cholesterol and blood pressure levels, and lower rates of obesity and diabetes.

How to Re-populate Your Gut with Healthy Bacteria

We are often lacking in the healthy bacteria we need. This is primarily because the foods we eat don't support the growth of friendly bacteria, and second, because many of the medications we so readily take kill them off. Thankfully, it is quite possible to repopulate your gut with these healthy bacteria. Eat yogurt, preferably plain and unsweetened, low-fat or non-fat, which contains live cultures. Greek yogurt has the highest level of these probiotics; kefir is another rich source of healthy bacteria. You should have at least 2 to 3 servings per week of these probiotic dairy foods such as Greek yogurt and kefir. Also include unsalted raw nuts like walnuts, almonds, or pecans and natural berries, like wild blueberries or fresh strawberries to your daily diet—these types of foods are loaded with the soluble fiber and other phytonutrients that promote healthy gut bacterial flora. Make this kind of breakfast a habit and you will create an ideal environment in your gastrointestinal tract that will trim your waistline, keep your heart and blood vessels soft, supple, and youthful, and your brain sharp and happy. If you don't like yogurt, you can take a probiotic supplement available at organic food stores.

Checklist for Cultivating Friendly Bacteria to Be Your Biological "Team You"

1. Eat at least 2 colorful vegetables and fruits at each of your 3 daily meals.

2. Consume probiotics (unsweetened yogurt, kefir, etc.) at least 3 times per week.

3. Eat at least 1 sulfur-containing vegetable (cabbage, kale, broccoli, Brussels sprouts) daily.

4. Drink 6 to 8 glasses of water daily.

5. Use 1 heaping tablespoon of sugar-free Metamucil in 16 ounces of water daily.

6. Eat garlic and onions regularly, and try to make sure your companions do too (so they won't notice your garlic-breath).

7. Avoid sugar, and anything made with grains. If you are at or near your ideal body weight, it is okay to eat up to 1 daily serving (one half cup cooked) of 1 of these 4 grains: wild rice, steel-cut oats, quinoa, or pearled barley.

CHAPTER 8

The Supreme Power of Diet

Eat Like a Mediterranean Peasant; Enjoy Regal Health for a Century

During a recent trip to southern Italy, Joan and I stayed in the little seaside village of Pioppi—the home of the Mediterranean diet. During the 1940s and 1950s Ancel Keys, a famous American nutritionist, lived with and studied the people of Pioppi. He came to the conclusion that among the various eating styles from around the world, the traditional cuisine of the people living on the shores of the Mediterranean Sea, especially in France, southern Italy, Crete, and Sardinia was a major reason for their remarkable health and longevity. Keys personally adopted this Mediterranean cuisine for his own diet, and went on to live for 102 years as one of the most notable scientists of the 20th century. This style of eating, which has been followed for centuries by the peasants of the Mediterranean region, seems to be especially effective for keeping the heart and brain youthful and for preventing diseases like diabetes and Alzheimer's.

On our trip we became friends with Luigi, a native of this region of Italy, who for an entire day took us up into the countryside to meet and dine with his friends: Maria Theresa and Frederico. They lived and worked on a family farm that has for centuries produced nearly all of the food and beverages that their family consumes. They have an olive grove and make their own extra-virgin olive oil each year. They also have grapevines and produce a delicious dry red table wine that we enjoyed during the time we spent with them. They grow tomatoes, eggplant, carrots, greens, onions, and garlic, all of which were part of the feast they prepared for us. We stopped at a local fish shop on our way to visit Maria Theresa and Frederico. We purchased mackerel and octopus that had been caught only 2 hours before, and was so fresh, it was still alive and had the salt-spray scent of the sea.

Traditionally, the Mediterranean diet included very little meat, because the poor people of this region could not afford it. Instead they ate fish, nuts, beans, and small amounts of cheese. Indeed, Frederico served us a modest portion of a low-fat soft white cheese that they made earlier that morning from the milk of their 2 dairy cows. While they milked the cows, Joan bonded with the month-old calf in the barn. We dressed our salad with olive oil and fresh juice from lemons picked from trees also growing on their land. Joan and I like to think of ourselves as connoisseurs of olive oil (at home in our household of 4, we go through over a liter of olive oil each week). Maria Theresa's delicious extra-virgin olive oil had a green tint and left a peppery burn at the back of the throat—evidence of very high levels of antioxidants—the potent age-defying, disease fighting compounds found in high quality olive oil. During our day at their farm, we drank water, coffee, and a couple glasses of red wine with dinner. The Mediterranean peasants of ages past who performed hard manual labor for hours each day ate moderate amounts of bread and pasta; today, most people lead more sedentary lives and thus are better off avoiding these fattening foods, or consuming them in only very limited quantities.

This diet is high in fiber, antioxidants, vitamins, and omega-3 and monounsaturated fats; and is low in saturated fat, processed foods, and sugar. Interestingly, the scientific studies looking at the Mediterranean eating style generally show that it is not 1 single component that makes this diet so healthy, but rather the constellation of foods and beverages, along with an active outdoor lifestyle and an emphasis on socializing with family and friends. During our leisurely meal that lasted almost 3 hours, we ate multiple small, tasty, and nutritious portions and bonded with our new Mediterranean friends. Afterwards, we strolled around the grounds and enjoyed the natural beauty of their land. The Mediterranean diet is delicious and can keep you healthy and happy for a century, as it did for Ancel Keys, the Minnesota boy who adopted this diet in middle age.

Essence of the Mediterranean Diet and Lifestyle

- Fresh vegetables with each meal.
- Fresh fish and legumes daily.
- Extra-virgin olive oil.
- Red wine in moderation.
- Fresh fruit for snacks and/or dessert.
- Fresh nuts and seeds.
- Small amounts of meat used to flavor dishes rather than as the main focus of the meal.
- Modest amounts of dairy, mostly unsweetened plain yogurt and low-fat cheese.
- Daily physical activity, much of it outdoors in the sunshine and fresh air.
- Emphasis on smaller serving sizes, fresh foods, and nutritional balance, with focus on pleasure, conversation and companionship during meals.

The Rules of the Diet

You want to feel great, think clearly, and enjoy life for almost a century? You are going to have to be very smart about what, where, and when you eat. The power of an ideal diet is unparalleled for rebuilding a healthier and more vigorous you. But let's be clear: you must consistently do 3 things: 1) eat and drink the right stuff, 2) strictly avoid the wrong stuff, and 3) don't eat for about 12 hours during the night time hours. This eating plan is tasty, fresh, and brimming with nutritious foods and drinks; it's low in caloric density, but high in fiber and will keep you energized and satisfied for hours. Your genome has been designed by evolution for hundreds of thousands of years to thrive with this diet and this pattern of letting your system purify itself for about 12 hours each night. Eating and drinking this way will completely change the way your genes work, and will create 'a whole new you.'

First and foremost, you must be eating a lot of fresh, colorful non-starchy vegetables, ideally at least 4 to 5 cups daily. Additionally, eat low-glycemic fruits like berries, apples, oranges, etc.; about 2 cups daily. Also, consume a healthy protein like fish (not fried), non-fat yogurt, black beans, eggs, skinless poultry, etc., with each of your 3 daily meals. Make sure your protein serving size is about the size of the palm or your hand. Fresh, lean red meat (grass-fed or game meat is ideal) is acceptable 2 or 3 times per week, but try to cook at low temperatures (ideally to not more than medium-rare). Include a modest amount of healthy fat in each meal, like nuts or seeds (a serving size is 1 small handful), extra-virgin olive oil, avocados, etc. For beverages choose mostly non-caloric options such as water, tea (green tea is best), and coffee (hold the cream and sugar). Low-sodium V8® juice is the only juice you should drink—it's a two-fer: you get fluids and it's like drinking your vegetables. Try to consume 1 or 2 servings of dairy daily, non-fat or low-fat (not more than 1 percent fat). If you are lactose intolerant, try coconut milk. If you can be disciplined about moderation, red wine, about 1 or 2 glasses, just before or with the evening meal can provide benefits to your health and well-being.

"If it came from a plant, eat it.
If it was made in a plant, don't eat it."
–Michael Pollan

Equally important as consuming the foods and drinks that make you thrive, is not consuming the foods and beverages that cause accelerated aging and chronic diseases. Let's make this simple and straightforward: consume almost nothing with added sugar, high-fructose corn syrup, or artificial sweeteners. The only exception we personally make is 1 tablespoon of artificially sweetened Metamucil each day. Also, largely avoid grains, especially processed grains. One small serving (one-half cup) once daily of wild rice, steel-cut oats, quinoa, or pearled barley is okay for most people. Eat and drink nothing made of wheat; even whole-wheat products are off limits. Make it your priority to consume things that are as close to their natural state as possible. Try to avoid foods and beverages that contain more than about 2 or 3 ingredients.

Don't believe the old urban myth that how many calories you consume is the only factor that determines your waistline. Recent studies refute that old idea that 'a calorie is a calorie.' We can now state confidently that not all calories have similar effects on metabolism (resting metabolic rate), appetite, cardiovascular risk factors, and weight. It should come as no surprise that the best kinds of calories are those that come from unprocessed, low-glycemic-index foods. So choose unprocessed whole natural foods whenever you can and cut back on high-glycemic-index foods like anything with concentrated or added sugars, and all processed grains including white bread, white rice, potato products, and prepared breakfast cereals.

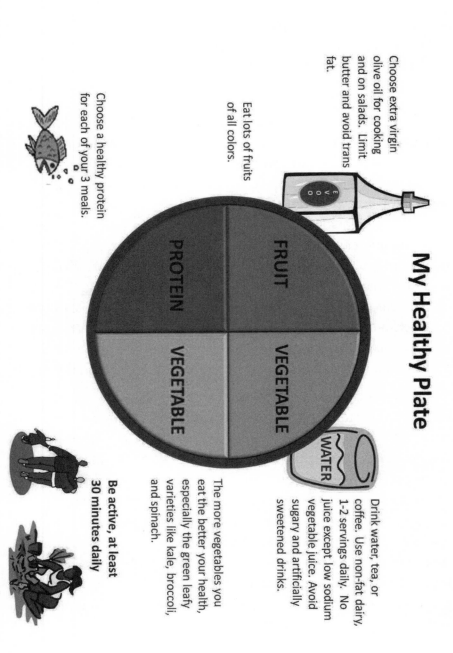

My Healthy Plate

Choose extra virgin olive oil for cooking and on salads. Limit butter and avoid trans fat.

Eat lots of fruits of all colors.

Choose a healthy protein for each of your 3 meals.

PROTEIN

FRUIT

VEGETABLE

VEGETABLE

WATER

Drink water, tea, or coffee. Use non-fat dairy, 1-2 servings daily. No juice except low sodium vegetable juice. Avoid sugary and artificially sweetened drinks.

The more vegetables you eat the better your health, especially the green leafy varieties like kale, broccoli, and spinach.

Be active, at least 30 minutes daily

You Are What You Eat

Don't Settle for Ordinary—Make Your Life Extraordinary!

Imagine being able to live for 100 years, and being mentally sharp, physically strong, and vigorous for the entire century. You wouldn't die slowly, wasting away over years or decades from horrible chronic incurable illnesses. Instead, you would live about 9 or 10 decades and then pass away rather quickly. Though this may seem like a pipe dream, it can be possible if you follow a gentle discipline where you eat foods as close to their natural forms as possible, and, like your ancient ancestors, exercise naturally, and relax deeply. You will also need to stay in close touch with your trusted doctors, and when necessary, employ the scientific marvels of cutting-edge, 21st century medicine.

Nutrition Revolution

We are on the verge of a revolution in health and medicine. Nutrition has been neglected, misrepresented, and abused. The ideal diet is finally becoming clear, and its power in health and healing is astounding. It is simple, practical, and sustainable for a lifetime. This diet (see "My Healthy Plate," left), especially when used in combination with daily exercise, will ensure vibrant and resilient good health for a lifetime. Getting smart about what you eat is an essential step for a strong, lean, and resilient body, and a sharp, focused, and cheerful mind. Embrace the nutrition revolution and you can thrive like never before. One of the most enlightened approaches to nutrition is detailed by Loren Cordain, PhD, in his extraordinary new book, *The Paleo Answer*. Loren is a friend and colleague; we have coauthored together 6 scientific articles published in medical journals over the past 8 years that describe benefits from following diet and exercise patterns consistent with our hunter-gatherer heritage. Dr. Cordain is the father of the Paleo Diet, which is the opposite of a fad diet. This is the pattern of eating nothing but wild plant and animal foods, and is what all of our ancestors did for millions of years. We are still genetically programmed to thrive best on this fare.

About 80 percent of your body composition—its shape, size, percent body fat, etc.—is determined by what you eat and drink. Most of the diseases you have or are likely to get are avoidable with an ideal diet. Do you want to continue to struggle with a snowballing mess of physical complaints, limitations, and chronic diseases, along with a less than ideal body, and a low-energy lifestyle? You must reject the toxic standard American eating habits, and tune out all the noise about fad diets for weight loss, and instead choose to feed your body the diet for which it was designed. The message is clear: real food direct from nature is wholesome and healing medicine; while highly-processed and refined food is tasty but toxic poison. The choice is yours—the stakes could not be higher.

Striking Changes in the Causes of Disease and Death

Only 2 or 3 generations ago, the principal agents of disease and death were microbes. Back when my great-grandfather, Henry O'Keefe, M.D., was making house calls on a horse-drawn sleigh in rural North Dakota, life expectancy was only 45, and most people died of infections like pneumonia and tuberculosis. Today, non-communicable diseases like heart disease, cancer, and diabetes usually kill us; and now the agents of disease are mostly self-inflicted.

Without question, many of the agents of disease and premature aging today are disguised as tasty treats in our diet. Most people understand that their diet and lifestyle might be problematic, but are confused about exactly where to find the villains that are causing them to be fat, tired, depressed, diabetic, or sick... or all of the above. In order to flourish and maintain a youthful mind and body for a century you need to avoid the agents of disease and embrace the foods that confer well-being. You may be surprised to discover the source of your health woes, and the natural cures.

Importantly, this is a 2-step cure: every day you have to consume the foods and beverages that bestow vitality, and do your best to avoid the agents of disease. Follow this plan and you will see amazing progress in virtually any health issue you may be struggling with today.

Agents of Disease

Excess Calories

We have patients who do well on the Weight-Watchers diet. Others have lost weight eating mostly fatty meats, cheese and cream. Yet others have shed excess pounds eating no fat. Whether vegan or Atkins, low-carb or low-fat, or whatever, most diets work, for a while anyway. The reason why you can lose pounds on any diet is that, one way or another, they all cut down on calories, which is a good thing because excess calories consumed is the number 1 problem with the American diet. One of Joan's clients, Bruce, told her, "I am following the Seafood Diet." She remarked, "Well it doesn't seem to be working; your weight is 5 pounds higher than when I saw you last. Tell me how this Seafood Diet works." Bruce replied, "It's simple—when I see food, I eat it!"

Over the past 30 years the daily average calorie consumption in the U.S. has increased by about an average of 400 calories, or 18 percent; this is the main reason why today 7 out of 10 of us are overweight or obese. And most of those added calories come from increased consumption of processed foods containing ingredients such as wheat, corn, and soybeans. Flour and cereal products account for about 40 percent of the total calorie increase; high-fructose corn syrup and other added sugars, typically in the form of sweetened drinks, are the other major source of new and extra calories. Sadly and tellingly, none of the large increase in calories during the past 3 decades has been due to fruits and vegetables—consumption of these has remained unchanged. A sure-fire method for dramatically improving the health and life expectancy of animals and humans is to reduce calorie intake to about the same as the calorie expenditure each day—this usually involves cutting daily calories by about 20 to 30 percent and increasing physical activity. You can count on this simple and potent strategy, to improve all of your cardiovascular risk factors like cholesterol, blood pressure, blood sugar, and waist size. And the best way to painlessly cut daily calorie intake: simply avoid processed foods, fried foods, and anything with added sugar or refined grains.

While you can lose weight by eating nothing but 1,200 calories of cheesecake a day, you will need to do more than cut calories to feel and see the full transformative power of optimal nutrition.

Grains (Especially Wheat), Starches, and Added Sugar

One of my patients asked, "Dr. O'Keefe, what can I do to lower my high triglycerides without resorting to medications?" So I told him, "You can start by strictly avoiding things that are white and/or sweet." He looked over at his loving, fair-skinned wife and smiled, "Honey, looks like you are off limits for me for the time being, at least while I get my triglycerides under control."

"Lose the wheat, lose the weight, and find your path back to health." That's the mantra of Dr. William Davis, cardiologist from Milwaukee and author of the brilliant best seller *Wheat Belly*. We are a nation of wheat-aholics. If you are like the average American, you consume 133 pounds of wheat per year, equivalent to about a half a loaf of bread per day. Add to that, the third of a pound of added sugar the average American consumes each day, and you have a recipe for disaster. The origins of this widespread wheat and sugar addiction and the ensuing obesity contagion can be traced back to 30 years ago when the U.S. Department of Agriculture began waging a propaganda campaign urging Americans to eat 6 to 11 servings of grain per day, and cut back on all fats. The result, according to Dr. Davis, is that today, if you are walking through a crowded international airport, the Americans can be easily identified by their characteristic wheat belly, or food-baby, or man-breasts, or love handles, or muffin-top. Call it death by food pyramid! Adding fuel to the fire is the fact that modern wheat has been genetically altered to be absorbed almost instantaneously after consumption, causing our blood sugar to spike, disturbing our hormones and causing cravings for more wheat and sugar. Wheat flour, for many people, is highly addictive because this roller coaster effect on blood sugar causes a vicious cycle of hunger and overeating, which consequently leads to inflammation, fatigue, obesity, depression, and disease.

One of our patients tried to convince us that doughnuts should qualify as health food because, after all, they are *hole* grain. But seriously, the notion that whole grains are good for us is an urban myth. Sure, whole wheat bread is better than white bread, but that's like arguing that cocaine is better for you than methamphetamine—you will be much healthier if you avoid both! Either whole wheat bread or white bread will spike your blood sugar worse than a candy bar or 2 tablespoons of pure sugar. In reality you would be better off avoiding all foods containing any wheat. Dr. Davis asserts that by eliminating all wheat products you can melt away excess belly fat, reduce inflammation and improve your overall health and vitality. We frequently recommend his book to our patients and are impressed by its effectiveness. Indeed, a growing scientific consensus suggests that eliminating wheat may dramatically reduce the odds of developing diabetes, Alzheimer's disease, heart attack, osteopenia (weak bones), arthritis pain, and many forms of cancer.

Take-home message: minimize intake of grains, especially anything and everything containing wheat, even whole grain wheat. Do not eat or drink anything with added sugar or high-fructose corn syrup. Man does not live by bread alone. The more bread you eat, the more bread you want. Truly, men and women would be much healthier and more attractive if they eliminated bread, in all forms, from their diet entirely. One of my patients asked me how I feel about all the delicious and convenient energy bars out there. I told him they are about the worst thing since sliced bread. Instead of bread or energy bars, eat your carbs in the form of non-fattening vegetables such as kale, spinach, and broccoli, and low-glycemic index fruits like berries, apples, and oranges. When you do eat grain, limit yourself to no more than 1 serving per day (one-half cup of cooked grains equals 1 serving). As we said earlier, the best choices are pearled barley, wild rice, steel-cut oats, and quinoa.

Excess Salt

Sodium (AKA salt), when consumed in amounts above about 1,500 mg daily, will raise blood pressure and cause heart attacks and stroke. Above 2,300 mg daily, sodium is a known carcinogen, predisposing especially to cancers of the gastrointestinal tract, such as stomach and colon cancer. Just because you shun the salt shaker doesn't mean you are good when it comes to sodium intake. More than 90 percent of the sodium in our diet comes from salt added to refined and processed foods—one more great reason to avoid the synthetic foods that are the standard fare today. As Jack LaLanne used to say, "If man made it, don't eat it!" Stick to foods and beverages as close to their natural forms as possible and you won't have to worry about how much sodium you're consuming. You can then add salt only to bring out flavor.

Excess Saturated Fat, Trans Fats

Try to avoid fatty meats, and stick with lean choices. When choosing dairy, non-fat is ideal, 1 percent is acceptable, too. Too much saturated fat, and almost any trans fats will raise your cholesterol and increase risks for diabetes, heart attack, stroke, and cardiovascular death.

Commonly Mistaken as Agents of Disease: These Are Not Evil Foods

Fats

Good fats, like the omega-3 oil in fish, and the unsaturated fats in nuts, extra virgin olive oil, and avocados, will help to keep you lean, youthful, and healthy. On the other hand, some fats, like the trans fats found in French fries and high levels of saturated fats present in fatty meats, ice cream, and butter, are among the worst things you can put in your mouth. So a low-fat diet isn't ideal, but neither is a high-fat diet if the fat is nasty pro-inflammatory, processed trans fats and excessive amounts of saturated fats. So, eat a diet rich in good fats, and low in bad fats. For the record, about 30 to 35 percent of your calories should come from fats, but less than 10 percent of the calories should be saturated fats; and eat virtually no trans fats.

Animal Products—Go for Vegetables, Not Vegetarianism

Crown Shakur, born in Atlanta, GA, died from malnutrition before his first birthday. His well-meaning vegan parents, who fed their newborn son mainly soy milk and apple juice, strictly avoided all food from animal sources. They were convicted of involuntary manslaughter for their child's death. Multiple such convictions of vegan parents have been handed down in American courts, highlighting the inescapable biological fact that humans are omnivores, and as such we need both plant and animal foods to survive.

America today is a land that indulges our freedom of choice. You can choose to have red hair and blue eyes, or to watch reruns of *Friends* and *Two and a Half Men* for 24 hours a day. For your morning coffee at Starbucks, you can choose to have a vanilla, half-caf, 1 percent, extra-hot, no-foam latte—but you can't yet choose your genes. Those genes, the blueprint your cells use to build and maintain you, specify the kinds of foods upon which you will either thrive or deteriorate. That's why not all diets are created equal, and why food cannot be like fashion fads that come and go.

Many vital nutrients, such as essential amino acids, DHA, vitamins B_{12}, A, and D, calcium and zinc are found predominantly in meat, fish, eggs, dairy, and other animal by-products. So, paradoxically, while fresh produce (vegetables and fruits) is the single most important component of a healthy diet, strict vegetarianism does not foster optimum human health. The traditional vegetarian diets, as in India, have always included eggs, dairy, and/or fish, which provided these nutrients.

Unfortunately, most animal-based foods in our modern diet are over-processed and unhealthy due to unnaturally high levels of saturated fats, sodium, nitrites, preservatives, and other additives, giving meat a bad reputation in many nutritional circles. Yet if you want a strong body, a sharp mind, and a powerful and vigilant immune system, you should try to consume a modest serving size of lean, healthy, fresh protein 2 or 3 times daily.

There is a lot of noise out there about the dangers of eating meat. And although I eat animal protein virtually every day, when I discuss this topic with my vegetarian friends and/or patients, I usually point out that I probably eat considerably more vegetables than they do. Dean Ornish will tell you being a vegan will cure heart disease. What he glosses over is the reality that if you eat no animal foods, you are at risk for brittle and broken bones, depression, Parkinson's disease, anemia, and some cancers. Steve Jobs, the heart and soul of Apple, was a strict vegan who sometimes ate nothing but apples and carrots for weeks at a time. He developed a rare type of pancreatic cancer that tragically ended his remarkable life in middle age. I have to believe that his eccentric diet, which was often woefully deficient in many essential nutrients, likely contributed to his cancer development at a relatively young age.

You are an omnivore—and you will be healthier in every way if you include animal foods in your diet on a daily basis. You just need to be very selective about the kinds of animal foods you eat. Excellent sources of high-quality protein are egg whites, whey protein, fish, seafood, low-fat poultry (skinless), and non-fat cottage cheese. When people say to me, "I'm surprised you eat red meat," I reply, "I'm okay with a modest-sized serving of red meat as long as it's very lean, and raw." Well, maybe not raw, but certainly not over-done or fried. Burning, blackening, frying, and over-cooking animal-based food creates cancer-causing chemicals. Lean red meat, especially game meats like venison (deer), and elk, can be highly nutritious, and tend to be very low in saturated fat.

Let's be clear, some of the most toxic foods in the American diet tend to be meat-based, like greasy cheeseburgers, fatty sausages, salty hot dogs, carcinogenic bacon strips, and chemical-laden deli-meats. But fresh, lean, medium-rare game meat, or grass-fed beef is highly nutritious, keeps you filled up for hours and helps you build muscle and rebuild tissue. You should eat a modest serving of protein with each of your 3 daily meals—especially breakfast. Non-fat, unsweetened plain Greek yogurt with raw unsalted almonds or pecans or walnuts, mixed with wild blueberries and/or strawberries is a perfectly delicious way to get your morning started off right with plenty of high-quality protein, calcium, probiotics, fiber, antioxidants, and potassium.

Dietary Cholesterol

Your blood cholesterol level is about 2 times as high as it was when you were born. In fact, you would be hard-pressed to find a wild animal on the planet with a cholesterol level anywhere near as high as the average modern human. And high cholesterol is one of the chief reasons most of us get clogged arteries as we age.

Yet many high-cholesterol foods such as shellfish, red meat, fish, eggs, and poultry can be very nutritious and do not raise your blood cholesterol nearly as much as foods high in saturated fat like butter, cheese, and deep-fried foods. So just because a food is high in cholesterol doesn't mean it's bad for you; and conversely, many of the worst foods like white flour, sugar, and trans fats contain no cholesterol.

LIST OF 20 TOP SUPERFOODS	
Leafy greens like kale, spinach, arugula, romaine	The single best superfood; full of age-defying, disease preventing nutrients.
Avocados	High in calories but loaded with anti-aging, disease-preventing nutrients.
Bell peppers	Green, orange, red, and yellow—eat them all.
Berries	Blackberries, blueberries, and strawberries: Mother Nature's candy.
Carrots	Get a healthy glow on your skin from the carotenoids.
Citrus fruits	Grapefruit, lemons, oranges, tangerines. All high in vitamin C and fiber. Don't drink orange or grapefruit juice—eat the whole fruit.
Cruciferous vegetables	Bok choy, Brussels sprouts, broccoli, cauliflower, cabbage, and kale. These sulfur-containing vegetables are uniquely powerful for preventing cancer. Try to eat at least 1 serving daily.
Eggs	No more than 1 yolk daily, but eat as many egg whites as you want.

Garlic and onions	Potent protection against cancer and heart disease.
Greek yogurt and kefir	Non-fat, plain, and unsweetened.
Green tea	Slows aging. Keeps mind sharp, focused, relaxed. Calorie-free.
Nuts	Almonds, brazil nuts, hazelnuts, macadamias, pecans, pepitas, and walnuts.
Extra virgin olive oil	Choose varieties that leave a peppery burn at the back of the throat after swallowing.
Coffee	Prevents diabetes, Parkinson's disease, depression. Calorie-free.
Red wine (white wine too)	One glass or 2 glasses with or before the evening meal is ideal.
Fish and seafood	Salmon, trout, shrimp, sardines, and herring. No fried fish.
Apples	Granny Smith and Red Delicious are highest in antioxidants.
Tomatoes	Eat with extra-virgin olive oil or fresh mozzarella cheese to improve absorption of nutrients such as lycopene.
Vegetable Juice	Low-sodium V8® juice is best.
Whey Protein	Mix in non-fat milk or coconut milk for an ideal post-workout recovery drink.

What We Actually Eat and Drink

People often ask us, "So what exactly do you eat?" We try to be conscientious about practicing what we preach, mostly because eating this way makes us feel good, think clearly, and look better.

From the time we awaken in the morning until about noon we each drink about 32 ounces of water, still or sparkling. When available, I add a fresh lemon slice to my water. We each drink another 32 ounces of water from noon until bedtime. During the morning, Joan drinks 2 cups of black coffee. I drink green tea, 3 to 6 cups throughout the day, but make a point to cut off the tea within 3 hours of bedtime. Joan drinks 1 glass of low-sodium V8® juice at lunch; I usually drink 2 glasses per day—1 at breakfast and 1 with my evening meal.

The Essence of a Balanced Diet

Protein Is Key

So let me be very clear about one point—protein is not optional. You need it 3 times each day. It is important to be picky about your protein and choose a healthy option such as egg whites, chicken or turkey breast, fish, lean red meat, whey protein, non-fat dairy, etc. For one of your meals you might try to choose vegetable protein such as nuts or legumes (beans, lentils, etc.). Portion size is important also. An ideal protein serving size is about the size of the palm of your hand, with a thickness about as wide as your little finger at the middle joint.

Protein is made up of large and complex molecules that take a long time to break down after a meal. That means your system slows digestion and delays emptying of the stomach as it works hard and long to absorb a protein meal. This keeps your blood sugar and triglycerides smooth and steady in the normal ranges. Additionally, a high-protein meal will keep you filled up much longer than typical easily digestible high-carb foods like French fries, white rice, candy, chips, etc. This is key because a meal high in protein and plant fibers prevents food cravings for up to 4 hours or more. If you are not hungry, it's easy to avoid eating trashy foods for snacks. But when you are starving hungry, you are at the mercy of every box of doughnuts, plate of cookies, drive-through, or vending machine you happen to come across during your day.

Fatty meats like full-fat hamburger and prime rib are off limits, as are over-processed meats like bacon and sausage. Jerky and deli meats, although often low in fat, are too high in salt and preservatives to eat on a daily basis.

Eggs: Healthy or Harmful?

Could eating eggs regularly be as harmful to your health as smoking?! A Canadian study published online July 31, 2012, in the journal *Atherosclerosis* reported this finding, though I have real doubts about the validity of their conclusions. These researchers sent questionnaires to 1,200 men and women (average age about 61) who were followed regularly in a preventive heart clinic. The study showed that regular egg yolk consumption was linked with plaque progression in the carotid (neck) arteries. Surprisingly, eating as few as 3 egg yolks per week seemed to predispose to an increase in plaque development. A larger and more impressive analysis of the egg dilemma came from the Physicians Health Study which has been following 21,300 male doctors for 20 years. This study found that men who ate 7 or more eggs per week were about 25 percent more likely to die from any cause compared to men who ate fewer than 7 eggs weekly. Importantly, 6 or fewer eggs per week was not linked with increased risk of heart trouble or death. The cardiovascular risk of eating eggs seems to be higher in diabetics, probably because they are at such high risk for arterial plaque development and thus are very sensitive to excess cholesterol in their diet.

Egg whites are a wonderfully healthy, clean and lean source of high-quality animal protein. Eating an egg white omelet with vegetables like tomatoes, spinach, mushrooms, and onions is about as nutritious as food gets. I personally don't miss the yolks at all, but if you do, try to limit yourself to not more than 3 yolks per week, and look for organic eggs that are high in omega-3 fats.

Father Jim is a friend and patient who raises chickens for eggs. I buy these natural brown eggs from him every chance I get. He treats his chickens as if they were his children. Just before dark each night, he goes outside and checks to see that they are all safely nestled into their roosts for the night. He worries about owls and other predators getting his beloved hens if they are left outside when darkness falls. If any of the birds have been chased up into the tree branches, Jim (a spry 75 year-old) props a tall ladder against the tree, and climbs up to rescue the stranded birds. He gently scoops up the chicken and shoos it into the safety of the chicken pen for the night.

To my vegan friends who shun all animal products because they cannot condone eating animals raised in inhumane conditions, I direct them to an egg producer like Father Jim. These eggs come from hens who are nurtured with tender loving care, have the run of acres of chicken paradise, and wander about during the day feeding on bugs and seeds and other natural food sources. His chickens are about as happy and healthy as birds can be, and their eggs are loaded with wholesome protein that is ideal for rebuilding the tissue in your body that is constantly being torn down in the course of day-to-day living. By including in your diet some wholesome animal protein, like fresh egg whites from free-range chickens, you will improve your health in many ways.

Color Your Life!

Second, you need to choose at least 2 colors (sorry, M&Ms® don't qualify) for each meal, including breakfast. This means eating 2 or more servings of plants, the fresher and more colorful the better—morning, noon, and night. As a rule, the healthiest thing you can put in your mouth grew in the dirt. Eating this much produce is not as tough as it sounds; 1 cup of strawberries (about 8 typical-sized berries) equals 2 servings of produce. Half of a grapefruit is a super-healthy component of any meal, plus it counts as 1 serving of fruit. Avoid fruit juices—they tend to spike your blood sugar (8 ounces of orange juice contains 24 grams of sugar, which is as much sugar as in 8 ounces of Coke). You are better off eating the whole fruit. If you are trying to lose weight, avoid fruit smoothies as well. These are high in calories and have most of the plant fiber ripped to shreds by the blender.

I explained to one of my female patients the importance of including a rainbow of colors in her diet: red strawberries and apples, oranges and carrots, yellow lemons, blueberries, green tea, or dark purple red wine (one glass), and so on. When I asked her how many colors were in the meal she cooked last night, she asked, "Does the black on the burned parts count as a color?" Um, no.

There is nothing like fresh produce for improving health and achieving weight loss. However, vegetables are more important than fruits, so try to work at least 1 vegetable into each of your meals. Vegetables are ideal for promoting fat loss and supercharging your health and vitality. I often have fresh avocado slices drizzled with fresh-squeezed lemon juice as part of my breakfast, or a glass of low-sodium V8® juice with a bowl of raw unsalted walnuts, almonds, or pecans with frozen wild blueberries. You will have no chance of hitting the 9 or more servings of vegetables and fruits per day if you don't start out by consuming at least 2 servings of produce at breakfast.

You need to eat breakfast every day—this signals your body to crank up its metabolism which will energize you. On the other hand skipping breakfast triggers hormonal changes that leave you feeling lethargic and hungry, and compels you to eat more calories throughout the day.

Leafy Greens

If you want to take 1 single step with your daily diet that will make it likely that you will be blessed with remarkably good health and extreme longevity, what would you guess that to be? The answer is a generous daily intake of raw or steamed leafy green vegetables.

When I was a kid, the only lettuce we had in our household was iceberg lettuce. When Joan and I were first married we ate romaine lettuce, then we moved to red leaf lettuce. But for the past 20 years, we have been huge fans of the real health and longevity stars of vegetation—leafy greens like baby spinach, kale, broccoli, and arugula. These are the most nutrient dense foods on the planet. Kale, a cross between cruciferous vegetable and a leafy green, may be the best of best (see the flat-belly salad recipe below).

A large meta-analysis of over 200 long-term observational studies concluded that raw vegetables showed a stronger protective effect against cancer than any other type of food. Leafy greens in particular also provide potent protection against macular degeneration—the leading cause of blindness in adults. Low carotenoid levels in the macula (the highly sensitive center of your field of vision where your visual acuity is the best) are a strong predictor of macular degeneration and blindness. If you can make sure you are eating leafy greens like kale and spinach at least 5 times weekly, your risk of developing macular degeneration falls by about 90 percent!

Joel Fuhrman, MD, advises his patients to tape a sign on their refrigerator door that says, "The salad is the main dish!" The base of your salad should be hearty greens like spinach or kale, not iceberg lettuce. Then add 2 more colors—your choice of red, green, or orange bell peppers, broccoli, carrots, onions, celery, mushrooms, snap peas, or whatever vegetables you enjoy. Be creative, indulge your vegetable passions, and dress it with extra-virgin olive oil and red wine vinegar or fresh lemon juice to enhance your body's ability to absorb the cornucopia of potent nutrients present in these vegetables. Now just add a modest serving of protein, like boiled peel-and-eat shrimp, or a chicken breast, and perhaps a bowl of raspberries for dessert, and you have a perfect meal.

Flat Belly Salad

This is a salad based we eat almost daily at the O'Keefe household. It is delicious, easy to prepare, and is healthier for you than any other food or dish on the planet. Unlike most other salads, this one also holds up well without wilting for 24 or 48 hours in the fridge, even with olive oil and vinegar on it. One of my favorite breakfasts is left-over Flat Belly Salad with a protein source like chicken breast, shrimp, or sardines.

<u>Flat Belly Salad</u>

- Kale
- Red, orange, green, and yellow peppers
- Purple cabbage
- Red onion
- Cilantro
- Dice up all the vegetables
- Toss salad with extra virgin olive oil and red wine vinegar

Easy as 1 – 2 – 3!

Okay, let's summarize: by eating a healthy protein* with each of your 3 daily meals, you will help to both control your hunger and keep your blood sugar in an ideal range, not too high or too low. This prevents your body from overproducing the free radicals that cause inflammation, premature aging and disease. By consuming at least 2 natural colors with each meal you are getting all sorts of disease-fighting, anti-aging nutrients that "rust-proof" your brain and body. So, with every meal think 1 – 2 – 3 (one protein*, 2 colors**, 3 times daily). By choosing good things first, you will be on your way to a whole new you.

* Protein foods: chicken, turkey, fish, shellfish, lean beef, pork, game meat, organ meats, egg whites, whey protein, nonfat cottage cheese, nuts, peanut butter, beans, lentils, tofu (for females only), low-fat cheese. A portion size is about the size of the palm of your hand, as thick as your little finger at the middle joint.

** Potatoes don't count as a vegetable. Sweet potatoes are ok. Potato skins (baked not fried) are acceptable.

We have a simple formula for eating. A few times a week, we go to Costco, Trader Joe's, and Hy-Vee (our local supermarket) so that we have plenty of fresh fruits and vegetables, along with fresh and frozen lean protein options. So meals never entail much planning. Below are meals from a random work week in our life.

Day	Meal Plan
Monday	Breakfast: Half a cup of berries. Scrambled eggs (using only half of the yolks and putting the other half of the yolks on the dog's food). Mix into the eggs diced tomatoes, green pepper, and onions. Lunch: Spinach salad topped with sliced chicken breast, (leftover from a dinner earlier this week) and sliced red bell pepper. Tossed with extra-virgin olive oil and red wine vinegar. 1 unsweetened grapefruit cup (slices). Dinner: Lemon Pepper Tilapia, baked. Salad with kale, shredded purple cabbage, red onions, and cilantro tossed with extra-virgin olive oil and fresh-squeezed lemon juice. Steamed broccoli, and ½ cup of wild rice.
Tuesday	Breakfast: 1 cup of unsweetened Greek yogurt mixed with a handful of nuts (like almonds, walnuts, pecans) and 1 cup of frozen mixed berries. Lunch: 8 oz. of skim milk mixed with chocolate whey protein (about 20 grams of protein) Fresh raw carrots, tomato slices. Dinner: Boiled shrimp, cooled on ice, dipped in homemade cocktail sauce (ketchup, horseradish, lemon juice mixed to taste). Brussels sprouts, brushed with olive oil, then baked. Kale salad (leftover from Monday's dinner.

Wednesday	Breakfast: I have Trader Joe's sardines, no added salt, packed in water. Fresh avocado slices with fresh lemon squeezed over it, 1 cup of fresh raspberries. Joan and the girls have fresh apple slices smeared with natural peanut butter and a bowl of fresh raspberries. Lunch: Salad of mixed spring greens with tomatoes, broccoli, and sunflower seeds, topped with cold shrimp and dressed with extra-virgin olive oil and balsamic vinegar. Dinner: Grilled sirloin steak (medium rare) with grilled asparagus. Arugula salad with extra-virgin olive oil and red wine vinegar. Baked potato skins, after baking scoop out and discard the whites of the potato. Brush with olive oil and sprinkle with Parmesan cheese, broil briefly.
Thursday	Breakfast: Steel-cut oats, 1 half cup, mixed with a handful of pecans, a few slices of banana and half cup of frozen wild blueberries (Wyman's Wild Blueberries from Costco). Lunch: Boar's Head low-sodium turkey slices, wrapped around 1 half of a fresh avocado cut in 4 slices. Wrap each slice of avocado in a slice of the turkey. 1 apple. Dinner: Baked pork chops on the bone. CCP salad (Cruciferous vegetable Cancer Prevention salad) including raw cauliflower, broccoli, green onions, and grape tomatoes mixed with extra-virgin olive oil dressing. Half a cup of watermelon for dessert.

Friday	Breakfast: Protein pancakes (6 egg whites, 1 cup non-fat cottage cheese, 1 cup of raw old-fashioned oatmeal. Blend in a blender, spray griddle with Pam cooking and cook slow on low-heat. Makes 16 silver-dollar sized pancakes). Serving size is 3 pancakes, smeared with peanut butter. Kiwi sliced (½ cup) and 1 small orange, cut into quarters.

Lunch: 1 cup of leftover CCP salad (even more delicious the second day). Scallops, 8 pieces, taken out of freezer, thawed and cooked in microwave. 1 cup of cantaloupe.

Dinner: Joan usually gets a break from cooking on Friday night. Our favorite takeout meal is salads from The Mixx, a salad restaurant. Joan usually gets a chopped salad of chicken, leafy greens and other vegetables. I get a salad of kale, radish slices, and quinoa topped with grilled salmon. |

The Fiber of Your Life!

I am a clinical cardiologist and Joan is a dietitian; we have a zeal for helping people regain and/or maintain their cardiovascular health and overall vitality; though honestly, neither of us have ever had much interest in doing animal studies. Over the past few months we unwittingly subjected our 3 dogs to a dietary experiment that we found enlightening. Coco, Joan's canine emotional supporter and biggest fan, is a cute and lovable mutt whose body had come to resemble an overstuffed sausage covered with curly hair. Even Brandon and Brady, my high-energy running partners, had put on a few stubborn pounds around their midsection, which made them look older and act less energetic.

So I found a new dog food that promises to get overweight dogs back to a healthy weight. It didn't take me long to figure out what the secret ingredient of this weight loss dog food was: fiber, and lots of it. I am in charge of poop patrol out in the back yard where the dogs run around, and immediately after switching to this new dog food I noticed that the amount of waste the dogs were putting out approximately doubled. And sure enough, over the next few months Brandon and Brady got their youthful waistlines back, and even Coco, though not quite svelte yet, was at least looking fitter than she has in years.

The latest and best science indicates that eating a high-fiber diet is one of the most important steps you can take for improving the health of your cardiovascular and digestive systems, as well as for promoting overall well-being and longevity. A recently published study shows that a high intake of plant fiber each day is even strongly linked to life expectancy. These researchers found that increased intake of plant fiber was associated with a lower risk of dying over a 9-year period compared to people who ate smaller quantities of fiber. Plant fiber, which is present in many foods including vegetables, fruits, berries, beans, nuts, and whole grains, helps the bowels move food efficiently through the digestive tract. A high-fiber diet helps prevent constipation, reduces blood levels of cholesterol and sugar, and may even lower risks of heart disease, diabetes, and some cancers. This new study from the National Institutes of Health involved about 390,000 adults and found that a diet rich in fiber from whole plant foods predicted longer lifespan. The individuals who were in the top one-fifth with respect to the quantity of fiber consumed each day were 22 percent less likely to die during follow up compared to people who were in the lowest one-fifth for daily fiber intake. The high-fiber intake was also associated with significant reductions in the risks of death from cardiovascular disease, infections, lung diseases, and some cancers. To get the impressive benefits noted in this study, women should eat at least 25 to 30 grams of fiber daily and men need to eat 35 or more grams of fiber daily. Tellingly, our ancient human ancestors living in the wild consumed at least 40 grams of fiber daily, so a high-fiber intake is the diet for which we are designed by nature.

Additionally, consider taking a soluble fiber supplement (like Metamucil) as part of your daily routine. Nuts are another good source of fiber. Studies show that eating nuts 5 or more times per week correlates with a 30 to 50 percent reduction in the risk of heart attack. Also, nuts like almonds, pecans, macadamia nuts, and walnuts are rich in many healthful nutrients like vitamin E, calcium, magnesium, and healthy fats. I personally eat raw unsalted nuts all day long and don't worry about the calories because I am very active and seem to have a high metabolic rate. Joan recommends that for an average American who is trying to lose weight, it's best to limit your intake of nuts to about 1 handful per day.

Eating Out Means Eating More

Researchers tracked about 1,000 people for a week, carefully documenting where and what they ate. What they discovered will not come as a shock: you are likely to eat many more calories when you dine in a restaurant rather than eating at home. Normal weight individuals, on average, consumed 550 calories during a meal at home versus 825 calories at a restaurant. Overweight or obese people consumed 625 calories at home compared to 900 calories when they ate in a restaurant. So when you eat out, you can expect to consume about 50 percent more calories than when you eat at home. What to do? It's simple, cook and eat at home more often; aim for at dining at home at least 14 meals per week. Harvard researchers have found that by eating more of your meals at home you are twice as likely to be successful in your efforts to lose excess weight, and you will save money to boot.

We eat breakfast and dinner at home almost 7 days per week. For our family, probably like yours, lunch for 5 days a week is by necessity, typically eaten at work or school. Yet even so, for lunch we routinely build our own large salad, and choose healthy vegetables, top it with a modest amount of lean protein, skip the croutons and fatty dressings and instead drizzle red wine vinegar and olive oil over our creation. In this way you can make your meal out as healthy as lunch at home. If you don't have access to a healthy salad bar, pack a lunch, and keep it simple, 1 protein and 2 or 3 colors.

Eating at home doesn't have to be time consuming or difficult. Joan is the queen of multi-tasking; while she is getting our dinner ready, she is often also running 2 small businesses and helping with homework. The key is to have plenty of healthy and easy options at home that are ready to prepare. Be flexible, and keep an open mind about eating different types of produce. You are aiming for about 10 servings a day of vegetables and fruit.

Breakfast: Your Most Important Meal

Upon awakening in the morning, the sunlight signals your brain that a new day has arrived. Similarly, breaking your nightly fast with a hearty meal of fresh produce and lean protein reinforces that message and synchronizes your body's circadian rhythms. The immediate changes in hormones deliver a jolt that jumpstarts your metabolism—revving up your engines to burn the fuel needed to energize your body and invigorate your mind.

Quench Your Thirst with Goodness!

Over the past 25 years, the average American has markedly increased the number of calories he or she drinks each day. During this same time period, the rates of obesity and diabetes have risen 3- to 4-fold, and experts believe that increased intake of high-calorie beverages is one of the major culprits making us fat. In fact today, beverages account for 21 percent of the total caloric intake. According to the Beverage Guidance Panel, the healthiest type of diet relies on natural, whole foods and not fluids to provide the vast majority of calories and nutrition.

Women need at least 72 ounces (9 cups) of fluid per day and men need approximately 100 ounces (12.5 cups) of fluid. If you are exercising vigorously, you will need even more. This need can be met almost entirely with water, although many people prefer to drink other forms of beverages. For the most part, we should be drinking calorie-free beverages (with no artificial sweeteners). Liquid calories should account for no more than 10 percent of your total daily caloric intake.

For example, if you are consuming a typical 2,000-calorie diet, you should make sure that not more than 200 of those calories are consumed in the form of beverages. Many Americans consume a large amount of sweetened beverages such as soda, which contain high fructose corn syrup. Downing 1 64-ounce Double Big Gulp from QuikTrip will immediately dump 900 inflammation-causing calories into your system.

Why a Coke a Day Might Make Your Doctor Dismay

Several studies have shown that drinking 1 or more soft drinks a day—even sugar-free artificially sweetened sodas—may increase your risk for obesity and diabetes.

One or more soft drinks per day heightens your risk of new-onset metabolic syndrome (pre-diabetes) by about 45 percent, regardless if it's regular or diet soda. Recent studies have reported that the consumption of 1 or more soft drinks daily is associated with:

- 31 percent greater risk of becoming obese, especially around the belly.

- 25 percent higher risk of having high levels of triglycerides or blood sugar.

- 32 percent higher risk of having low HDL cholesterol levels (the protective cholesterol).

- 74 percent higher risk of gout (a painful form of inflammatory arthritis).

One of the likely culprits in the sweetened drinks is high fructose corn syrup (HFCS). This very sweet but toxic substance is the darling of the processed food industry. HFCS increases triglyceride levels, causes inflammation, and has been linked to diabetes and heart disease. Even artificially sweetened sodas are corrosive to your health; a habit of 1 or more diet sodas daily has been linked to a 50 percent higher risk of stroke, heart attack and cardiovascular death over the course of a decade among the 2,500 people in the NOMAS (North Manhattan) Study.

So, what should you be drinking? The following is a list of healthy beverages. Anything not on this list probably should be avoided.

1. Water

2. Sparkling water (try adding a slice of lemon or lime to the beverage). Some of the habit-forming nature of Coke and other sweetened sodas is due to the carbonation that causes a burning / stinging sensation at the back of your throat and tongue. Those harmless CO_2 bubbles, just like jalapeno peppers, can be addictive because that burning feeling on the oral mucosal surfaces raises your blood levels of feel-good endorphins. Our family goes through about a case of flavored (unsweetened) carbonated water per week. La Croix, our favorite sparkling water, is free of calories, sodium, sweeteners, and anything artificial. It's delicious taste comes from natural flavors. We have come to crave these unsweetened throat-buzzing / tongue-stinging beverages.

3. Green tea (or any unsweetened tea)

4. Coffee (black or with skim or low fat milk)

5. Skim or 1 percent milk

6. Coconut milk, unsweetened (with added calcium)

7. Low-sodium tomato juice or vegetable juice, such as low-sodium V8®

8. Alcohol-containing beverages (unsweetened). These should be consumed only in light to moderate amounts, or they should be avoided altogether. One glass of red wine before or during the evening meal is ideal, although other drinks are acceptable as long as you keep it to just 1, never more than 2 a day.

The Only Juice You Should Ever Drink

A word of caution about heavily marketed antioxidant juice products touting overblown health benefits. These products, typically distributed via pyramid marketing schemes, are usually very expensive and despite their claims, do not provide health in a bottle.

A large recent study found that while consumption of fruits reduced risk of colon cancer, fruit juices were, in contrast, associated with increased risk of colon cancer. The only juice we heartily endorse is low-sodium V8® juice. An 8-ounce glass counts as 2 servings of vegetables. Loaded with potassium and rich in vitamin C and carotenoids, this is a beverage that is chock full of anti-aging nutrients, and it's also a terrific weight loss tool. Low-sodium V8® makes a great afternoon snack as well.

Get in the habit of having a glass of low-sodium V8® juice at breakfast. This should be a staple around your household. Just 8 ounces of low-sodium V8® is a quick and easy way to get 2 servings of vegetables before you leave the house to start your day. A recent study showed that drinking at least 1 glass of low-sodium vegetable juice daily can help overweight people with pre-diabetes lose their excess weight. This study from the Baylor College of Medicine found that study volunteers who drank at least 8 ounces of low-sodium vegetable juice as part of a calorie-controlled diet, lost 4 pounds over 3 months. Those who followed the same diet but drank no low-sodium V8® juice lost just 1 pound.

Seven out of 10 American adults fall short of recommendations, and over 90 percent of us do not achieve the 9 or more servings of vegetables and fruits that we advise. By drinking a glass of low-sodium V8® juice, you will increase your intake of vitamin C (125 percent of its Daily Value in just 8 ounces) and potassium (a whopping 820 mg of this blood pressure-lowering nutrient). Dress it up with a celery stick or a squeeze of fresh lime juice, or even a dash of pepper. This is an easy and delicious habit to help keep you lean and healthy. Make sure to use only the low-sodium vegetable juices. The regular V8® juice, for example, has about half of your allowance for sodium for an entire day in a single cup. If you prefer to make your own juice, do so from vegetables; fruit juice even if you make it yourself is too high in sugar.

The Dark Side of Soy

John was always a healthy, vigorous guy who began to notice some strange and worrisome symptoms. His breasts seemed to be enlarging, becoming swollen and painful especially just underneath his nipples. His sexual desire and performance were flagging for no apparent reason, and the growth of his beard slowed. When his doctors looked into John's complaints they discovered that his estrogen levels were off the scale—8 times higher than normal for an adult male, higher even than the levels seen in healthy young women. These bizarre hormonal levels were confirmed in a long and detailed series of medical tests, but no causes could be uncovered. Finally, one enlightened physician took the time to ask him about his diet and learned that because John had developed lactose intolerance in recent years he switched over to soy milk—in a big way. He was consuming 3 quarts daily of soy milk. He stopped all soy consumption immediately after his physician suggested that the soy phyto-estrogens were likely the cause for his mysterious health problems. Shortly thereafter, all of his complaints vanished over the course of a few weeks, and his hormones returned to healthy ranges.

Over the past 15 years, soy foods have come to be considered by many Americans to be among the healthiest of foods. Accordingly, consumption of soy has risen by 800 percent during this time period. In 1999, the FDA granted soy the highly coveted right to claim that a diet high in soy protein might reduce cholesterol and the risk of heart disease. Countless experts have recommended soy products such as tofu, soy burgers, soy cheese, edamame, etc., as a vegetarian substitute for meat. And millions of people forgo dairy to drink soy milk instead, thinking it will be better for their long term health.

However, we have been puzzled and concerned about several scientific findings regarding soy in recent years. Soy foods contain potent phyto-chemicals that have estrogen-like effects that can, when consumed in large quantities, disrupt the healthy levels of sex hormones, particularly in males. Animal studies show that males, when fed a diet high in soy, tend to become more irritable, which is a common symptom in males with low testosterone levels. Even more concerning is research suggesting that men who consume a relatively large amount of soy are at higher risk of developing Alzheimer's disease.

Recently, studies show that infants and children fed a high soy diet may have impaired immune systems predisposing them to allergies and asthma. The health ministries of several countries including Israel, New Zealand, France, England, Canada, and Australia recommended that soy products be avoided in infants and used sparingly in children due to concerns about possible problems related to growth, immunity, and hormonal levels. This means that soy protein is vastly inferior to lean fresh animal protein for building muscle, repairing tissues and providing the building blocks that are needed by your body to continually make new cells for rapidly turning over organs like the immune system, skin, and gastro-intestinal tract.

Bottom line, we think soy should be consumed only in moderation: not more than 2 or 3 servings per *week* in men and not more than 1 or 2 servings per *day* in women. You still need animal protein even if you do not like the idea of having to kill animals to provide for your food. So if you are vegetarian, make sure you eat 2 or 3 daily servings of fish, egg whites, or low fat or non-fat dairy, like nonfat unsweetened plain Greek yogurt, cottage cheese, or whey protein.

How to Deal with Emotional Eating

It is not just about what you eat, but why. So many of us overeat or make poor food choices as a response to emotions. We have a few ideas to help you avoid emotional eating. If you have an uncontrollable craving for an unhealthy food and you just have to have it, don't ruin your entire day; use Joan's 3-bite rule. Whatever it is you can't resist, take 3 bites, then stop and have a conversation with yourself. "You've tasted it; you've satisfied your craving, but you don't want to sabotage your weight loss for the day."

For many people, giving up comfort foods completely is emotionally difficult. But at least try to be moderate when you do give in to the urge to splurge. Keep in mind that emotional eating tends to occur when you are bored, procrastinating, happy, or sad. Whether you choose a candy bar when you are lonely or a doughnut when you are depressed, coming to recognize and control emotional eating is essential to successful weight management for many people. Stop and identify the emotion.

If you do feel compelled to eat when you aren't hungry, find a healthy comfort food instead of junk food. For example, an ounce of dark chocolate has redeeming value because of its antioxidant and healthy fat content; although many chocoholics have a hard time eating just a little chocolate. Better yet, have a cup of unsweetened hot or iced tea, a bottle of water, or a glass of sparkling water with a twist of fresh lime or lemon.

Fewer Food Choices: The Answer to Your Weight Problem?

The variety effect in humans and other mammals is partially explained by the fact that we seem to prefer food that differs from what we just ate. So it is clear that fewer choices in food on a day-to-day basis would be helpful in keeping weight under control. How to make this happen is a more problematic issue. One effective way to reduce variety is to consider major types of foods—for example, highly processed ones and those containing trans fats, high fructose corn syrup, wheat, sugar, or white flour—should be strictly off-limits. If you can discipline yourself to think this way, you will automatically eliminate many foods, particularly the unhealthy ones that you are likely to have access to in your daily routine.

Four Little Words That Can Change Your Life

"I don't eat that." Get used to repeating this phrase, as often as you need to, whether it is to yourself, or to someone offering you one of the delicious but toxic treats that seem to be everywhere. Doughnuts, milk shakes, and other sweetened drinks, fries, candy bars, cheeseburgers, breakfast cereals, cakes, pies, cookies, chips, crackers, and the like. When Joan and I see treats like these we don't think about how good they would taste, we think about how uncomfortable we would feel about an hour later. With time, "I don't eat that" will become a deeply ingrained habitual response, and these sorts of foods and drinks will start to seem virtually inedible to you.

A recent study found that 4 out of 5 people who were taught to use the phrase "I don't eat that" when faced with a tantalizing but unwholesome treat were able to stick to their healthy eating habits. In contrast, only 10 percent of the people who used other phrases like "I can't eat that" were able to stick with their diet. You will find that declaring, "I don't eat that" to yourself and to the world is empowering, and puts you back in control. By saying, "I can't," you are implying you are depriving yourself by giving up something desirable.

Snacks: Only If You Are Truly Hungry

If you eat a high protein, high fiber, straight from nature breakfast, you probably won't be hungry all morning and should be fine until lunch. But many people start having problems sometime after lunch. The stress, boredom, unhappiness, and the like start setting in for many people by midafternoon. Ask yourself, "Am I feeling that gnawing hunger feeling in my belly?" If the answer is no, choose to do something else, like have a bottle of water or a cup of coffee or green tea, or get up from your desk and go for a walk, even a short stroll, ideally outside, perhaps while you call a friend or family member, or even climb up and down a few flights of stairs. If the answer is yes, you do sense a gnawing feeling in your tummy, choose a smart snack—and keep it to no more than 200 calories. You want a natural combo of fiber to keep you full, fresh produce for an instant energy boost, and protein for lasting satiety and muscle building. For an ideal snack, Joan recommends 1 color (a brightly-hued vegetable or fruit) and 1 protein. Examples of a healthy snack for those times when you are truly hungry:

- One hard-boiled egg with ½ of a banana.

- One pear (including skin) with 3 slices of turkey breast.

- A glass or can of low-sodium V8® juice (freshen it up with a squeeze of lime, over ice, maybe even with a stalk of celery), and a handful of nuts. The right serving size for nuts is a handful, just make sure you can close your fist around the nuts.

- Apple slices smeared with peanut butter (1 tablespoon).

- Carrots (½ cup) dipped in hummus (1 or 2 tablespoons).

- Grapes (12) and 1 cheese stick (2 percent mozzarella).

- Cup of unsweetened sparkling water or iced tea with a twist of fresh lemon, and a small serving of nuts (1/8 cup).

- Cup of green tea with non-fat, unsweetened Greek yogurt, (4 to 6 ounces, mix in a few berries or raw nuts).

For a special treat with redeeming nutritional qualities try a few dark chocolate-covered almonds or blueberries. Still, you will need to be prudent about serving size, as these are very high in calories. So limit your intake to about an ounce (about 120 calories worth), which is about 8 chocolate covered almonds or 10 chocolate covered blueberries. Dark chocolate covered espresso coffee beans are an energy-boosting snack that is also a rich source of anti-aging, disease fighting antioxidants. But be careful about treating yourself to these kinds of sweet but healthy snacks like dark chocolate, as they will often stimulate your appetite for more sweets and may halt your weight loss for the day. In fact if your plan is to lose weight, we can incorporate these dark chocolate covered treats later, but for now you should avoid them altogether. And even if you are at ideal weight and burning a lot of calories exercising every day, you may want to limit these snacks to just once or twice per week. Chocolate, like many other intense but addictive pleasures in life, can be a slippery slope for susceptible individuals. Most of us have at least one weakness where abstinence is easier and more successful than moderation.

Become a Health-Nut

Nuts are good for you—really good for you as it turns out. On a daily basis, you ought to be eating about a handful of nuts (ideally raw, unsalted nuts). Nuts are among nature's top sources of disease-fighting, anti-aging nutrients. These naturally tasty treats are high in fiber, antioxidants, healthy plant protein, and beneficial fats.

My mother, Leatrice, now 83, looks and acts decades younger than her age. Throughout her life, nuts have been her favorite food. Leatrice eats nuts every single day, and has to limit her nut intake at happy hour or it blunts her appetite for dinner. I am convinced that her generous consumption of nuts has played a central role in keeping her skin, brain, and heart so youthful. The monounsaturated and polyunsaturated fats that are abundant in nuts (and avocados, olive oil, and pumpkin seeds) are essential for waterproofing your skin. This attribute of becoming 'like water off a duck's back' ensures your that your skin stays plump, hydrated, and radiant looking. We love to visit Mediterranean shores, and are always impressed by the soft supple-looking skin of handsome and beautiful Italians who are famous for their daily intake of olive oil. A large study of women found that those who ate several servings of nuts weekly had an astounding 74 percent lower risk of cardio-vascular disease, such as heart attack and stroke. Other studies show that regular consumption of nuts will lower your chances of developing Alzheimer's disease, diabetes, and breast cancer.

Walnuts are highest in the beneficial omega-3 fats, and pecans are loaded with antioxidants. Brazil nuts are the single best dietary source of selenium—a powerful mineral for warding off chronic diseases like diabetes. Almonds are especially high in fiber and calcium and have been shown to lower cholesterol and blood sugar. Pistachios are rich in antioxidants and raise your good or HDL cholesterol, while sunflower seeds help to lower bad choles-terol. Among the nuts, chestnuts are lowest in calories and fat, yet high in fiber. Cashews are rich in copper and zinc, but not quite as healthy as other nuts. Peanuts are actually a legume not a nut, so the health benefits of peanuts do not measure up to the tree nuts mentioned above. Still, lightly salted peanuts are okay as an occasional snack (say when you are trapped in the middle seat of a crowded commercial airliner). Natural peanut butter dabbed on banana slices is a favorite on the O'Keefe breakfast menu.

Nuts are high in calories, so if you have a weight issue you need to be careful about sticking to about 1 serving (approximately 1/8 to 1/4 cup) of nuts per day. However studies show that people who eat 2 or more servings per week actually have lower rates of obesity than those who rarely eat nuts. A serving of nuts will increase satiety for hours, preventing cravings for junky snacks and thus may help prevent overeating. Shoot for about 1 small handful of mixed nuts daily, preferably unsalted or lightly salted. If you are an athlete and are burning a large number of calories by exercising vigorously, nuts are a great way to increase your intake of healthy calories. If you are underweight and need to regain strength and a few pounds, nuts are a wonderful solution.

CHAPTER 9

Silent Stalkers

How Spikes in Blood Glucose and Fats Cause Inflammation, Aging, and Disease

Try This at Home

This year Caroline, our 13-year-old daughter, was regularly assigned a *My Own Science* project by her seventh grade science teacher. For one of these little home experiments we decided to see how her system responded to different meals by checking her blood sugar with a home glucometer before and after eating. Joan prepared a 450 to 500-calorie, high-protein breakfast of scrambled eggs, lean ham, mixed berries, and a glass of skim milk. Caroline gobbled this down and her blood glucose didn't budge: she had a fasting morning reading of 82 that fell to 80 when we re-measured her glucose 90 minutes after breakfast. All morning long she was cooperative, sweet, happy, gentle, and energetic... and not hungry.

For lunch, Caroline had a very different meal (though it contained the same number of calories as breakfast), consuming a large bowl of white rice dressed with some soy sauce. She drank 16 ounces of a fruit punch. Her blood sugar started at 75 and surged to 125 an hour and a half later! During the first hour after lunch she was wired on a sugar high, but then as her blood glucose plummeted she quickly morphed into the Wicked Witch of the West arguing with her siblings, slamming doors, being uncooperative with us, and eventually needing of a nap. Dinner was a typical O'Keefe-style meal: grilled salmon, spinach salad with cherry tomatoes dressed with extra virgin olive oil and lemon juice, steamed broccoli, and fresh pineapple for dessert. This meal, also 450 to 500 calories, barely raised Caroline's blood glucose from 79 to 85.

We encourage you to try this experiment on your own. Home glucometers are inexpensive and easy to use. You will be astounded at the drastic differences in your blood sugar readings depending on what you choose to consume. It is a great way to drive home the primary concepts of a healthy, balanced diet. Keep in mind Caroline is a very fit and healthy, lean and active, teenager. Her system is about as good as it gets for efficiency in clearing sugar from the bloodstream, and still she had a dangerously high spike in blood glucose after a single meal of white rice and high-fructose corn syrup. Your system is probably much less adept at the fundamentally important process of keeping your blood glucose in an optimal range.

The One and Only You

You are unique—1 in 7 billion to be precise. The singular combination of your specific set of genes influenced by your lifestyle, diet, attitude, and environment determines exactly who and what you are. This means that we each have our individual strengths and weaknesses. Chronic inflammation is the common denominator behind about 80 percent of the diseases that zap our vitality, ravage our health, and eventually kill us. Inflammation will seek out and attack you at your most vulnerable spots. If you pay close attention to how you feel after eating a high-calorie junk food meal, like a large cheeseburger with fries and a Coke, especially if you also happen to be stressed or sleep deprived, you can pick up clues about some of your weak spots.

For our teenage children, when they eat junk food the inflammation shows up on their face as acne about within a day after the dietary indiscretion. My patient, Kelsey, complained to me about soreness and redness in the arthritic joints in her hands. She would notice this about an hour or 2 after over-indulging in sugary or starchy foods. She also had inflamed plaques festering silently in her coronary arteries that she couldn't feel until she had a heart attack at age 55. For many people, including Joan, the sluggishness, mental fog, and fatigue that set in after a large, unhealthy meal are signs that the brain is under siege and bogging down from a flood of free radicals generated by too much sugar and fat.

The #1 Secret to Slow Aging and Prevent Disease

Hang with me for a moment as I explain a somewhat complex concept. If you can grasp this idea and deploy its strategies, it will revolutionize your life. You are probably oblivious to the most important factor determining the health of your diet. After a meal, dangerously elevated levels of glucose and triglycerides (fats) in your bloodstream fly under your conscious radar, and although they usually go undetected, these resulting spikes can eventually wreak havoc on your health and longevity.

All of the energy necessary for you to move, to think, to grow, and to stay alive comes from your metabolic engine—which resides collectively within the mitochondria—the microscopic power generators, within each of your 10 trillion cells. Those little mitochondrial furnaces burn only 2 fuels—glucose and fatty acids. The smoke that comes off from that metabolic fire consists of free radicals or pro-oxidants that, if not neutralized, will cause you to rust from the inside out, so to speak, leading to premature aging and disease.

Your system is a machine that will run smoothly and efficiently when you feed it the fuel for which it has been designed by nature. However, just like throwing too much wood and kindling on a fire all at once will make it burn out of control causing toxic amounts of smoke to billow through the air, the metabolic smoke from eating a high-calorie, fast food meal will billow through your cells, tissues and organs, polluting your system. After you gulp down a large plate of spaghetti and cheesecake for dessert, this massive slug of calories is digested almost immediately, leading to dramatic spikes in your blood sugar and fats. This fuel floods your engine, causing the metabolic fires to churn out massive amounts of smoke in the form of free radicals like super-oxide anions. These toxic molecules oxidize your DNA which leads to premature aging and cancer, and oxidize your blood cholesterol, which leads to inflammation and disease in your arteries, heart, and brain. Additionally, these spikes in glucose trigger corresponding spikes in insulin, which directs your body to store a lot of those extra calories as belly fat. In turn, this causes a downward spiral because excess abdominal fat churns out inflammation and leads to hormonal disruptions that predispose to even higher spikes in glucose and triglycerides after eating.

Contrast that to what happens after a meal consisting of steamed broccoli, a salad of kale and shredded red cabbage drizzled with extra virgin olive oil and vinegar, a modest serving of lean protein (skinless chicken breast or baked fish for example), with water and/or tea for your beverage, and blackberries for dessert. For starters, this straight-from-nature food is going to take much longer to eat than processed food because you are going to have to do a lot more natural food-processing (chewing) yourself, and an even longer time to digest. The calories from this meal will trickle into your bloodstream never causing your blood glucose or blood triglycerides to rise above 100, and your metabolic engine will burn those calories cleanly as they arrive, rather than storing them in belly fat. Furthermore, all of those natural pigments from the colorful plants are antioxidants that will bind to and neutralize the oxidants (smoke) thrown off by your engine as it burns the glucose and fats from the meal.

A study by Dr. Robert Vogel showed that the blood vessel function will deteriorate by about 50 percent within 2 hours after a junk food meal even in healthy young volunteers. Practically speaking this means that the arteries constrict when they should be dilating, and they lose their Teflon-like non-stick lining that prevents abnormal clotting. Although this post-meal stress settles down by 4 to 6 hours, the typical 21st century American overloads their system with excessive calories from sweet, fatty, and/or starchy treats 3, 4, 5, or more times each day; leaving their blood vessels under constant siege. Like waves crashing against a shore, this destructive process can eventually erode your health and vitality by filling your arteries with inflamed plaques and jeopardizing the well-being of your heart and brain.

How well your body metabolizes food is a major predictor of your long term vigor, mental clarity, physical strength, and life expectancy. In scientific papers in the *American Journal of Cardiology* and the *Journal of the American College of Cardiology*, we presented data showing that post-meal surges in the blood sugars and fats can lead to diabetes, heart disease, stroke, Alzheimer's disease and osteoporosis.

One of the scariest aspects of this post-meal stress is that it usually remains completely hidden. Traditionally we only measure glucose, cholesterol, and triglycerides in the fasting state (at least 12 hours since last intake of calories). Ironically, about the only time most people ever fast is when they come in to have their cholesterol and glucose checked. Virtually the rest of their waking lives they are in the postprandial (or post-eating) condition which could be silently ravaging their cardiovascular system.

This post-meal stress is a chronic problem for a large proportion of Americans. A steady diet of processed, high calorie foods creates a vicious cycle, causing immediate inflammation and stress, and over time leading to weight gain. Excess belly fat aggravates the tendency for the blood sugar and fats to spike after eating or drinking. Repeated meal-induced oxidative stress causes the blood pressure to rise and damages the pancreas predisposing to diabetes. Today about 1/3 of adult Americans have diabetes or pre-diabetes, yet most are unaware of it. A recent study showed that pre-diabetes even afflicts about 11 percent of teenagers (which translates to about 3 million American teens). This is a major reason why today's kids are on a trajectory to be the first generation in modern history to have a shorter lifespan than their parents.

Our ancient ancestors often lived on the edge of starvation, and we are genetically designed to thrive on low calorie, natural food that usually required strenuous hunting and gathering efforts to procure. In stark contrast, today we live in a world with delicious, cheap, and ever-present fast food, physically inactive occupations, and seated entertainment options. This mismatch between the world we are designed for and the one in which we live today is the genesis of most of the modern health woes, including the post-meal spikes in sugar and fat.

A healthy fasting glucose is less than 100; 100 to 125 is pre-diabetes and 2 or more fasting readings above 126 is diabetes. But you can have a normal fasting glucose of 90 and still have a level of over 200 an hour or 2 after eating. This latter number, the postprandial glucose, is the more important risk factor. An ideal glucose level 2 hours after consuming a meal is less than 120; a glucose of 140 to 200 is pre-diabetes and a level of 200 or higher is considered diabetes. It's easy to do this on your own by simply measuring your blood sugar about 1 or 2 hours after eating. Monitoring your blood sugars at home is a great way for you to see the striking hour-to-hour benefits of consuming a healthy diet and leading a physically active lifestyle. For example, a vigorous bout of aerobic exercise of 30 to 60 minutes done within a few hours of eating will lower the post-meal glucose surge by up to 40 percent.

Although your body's metabolism is mind-bogglingly complex and breathtakingly intelligent in its design and function, it can be simplified down to a practical take-home message: your machine will run best when you feed it only the natural fuel for which it's designed. Fill the gas tank of your car with jet fuel and it will run poorly, and eventually this high-octane kerosene will ruin the engine. Eating modern, refined, processed, high-calorie foods will do the same to your body. I cannot overemphasize the funda-mental and critical importance of this concept—if you want to stay youthful and healthy, you must avoid these post-meal spikes in glucose and fats. And the strategy to do that will sound familiar:

eat only whole, natural foods (that contain no more than 2 or 3 ingredients), balance your calories consumed with calories burned each day, keep your waist size to half your height in inches, exercise daily, and get 7½ to 9 hours of sleep each night.

The Anti-inflammatory Diet That Prevents Blood Sugar Spikes

Lean protein sources such as whey protein, egg whites, fish, and skinless poultry also blunt the post-meal spikes in blood sugar. These types of clean protein slow digestion by delaying stomach emptying. They also bolster your immunity and provide the building blocks to grow and repair tissue; but importantly they aren't loaded with saturated fats and/or carcinogens like those found in fatty burned red meats, or highly processed meats. Other great foods for preventing blood sugar surges after eating include nuts (tree nuts), and vinegar (which was used to treat diabetes before we had medications to lower blood sugar). One, or at the most 2, alcoholic drinks daily (ideally with or immediately before the evening meal) can help to blunt post-meal blood sugar spikes and lower the risk of developing diabetes by about 30 percent.

In short, the ideal diet for preventing dangerous blood sugar spikes is the same diet that has been consumed for centuries by the world's longest lived, healthiest populations from places like Okinawa and the Mediterranean. Plenty of vegetables, olive oil and vinegar, legumes, nuts, berries, fish, tea, water, and a modest daily dose of alcohol are the diet for both longevity and preventing diabetes. For countless generations the Okinawans have also passed down the 80 percent rule: eat only until you are about 80 percent full. You can overwhelm your system and cause blood glucose spikes by overeating even so-called healthy foods like fruits, whole grains, and legumes, so you have to practice portion control. You also might consider skipping a meal occasionally, like lunch for example. Sometimes instead of a sit-down meal over the noon hour, get out for a walk. When you get back, have just a quick snack, like an apple with a handful of nuts and bottle of water. This will give your system a much-needed break from the constant barrage of excess calories, allowing it to clean the sludge and clear the inflammation from your bloodstream.

The triglyceride level is lowest in the morning before you eat anything. A post-meal spike in triglycerides is also detrimental to the health of the arteries and heart. Omega-3 fat, in the form of fish oil, is very effective at reducing the post-meal triglyceride rise. Omega-3 improves cardiovascular and overall health in many ways, including reducing risks of sudden death, heart attack, and stroke. The dose of omega-3 for reducing triglycerides is larger, typically requiring 4 to 12 capsules daily (2,000 to 4,000 mg of EPA + DHA daily).

We have a growing list of medications that effectively normalize the post-meal blood glucose and lipid levels. Some of these are new, such as Januvia, Onglyza, Victoza, and Byetta, and have shown very promising results not only for normalizing glucose but also preventing heart attack and other cardiovascular problems. We believe that this new focus on identifying and treating the post-meal glucose and lipid levels will help to transform the long term health outlook for the growing numbers of Americans.

A Man Ahead of His Time

Weston Price, born in 1870, was a man who was way ahead of his time. Dr. Price was a dentist from Cleveland, Ohio, who figured out what was the matter with America's health decades before the average American even knew he or she had a health problem. Dental problems, much like heart disease, became so common during the 20th century that the general public seemed to accept them as part of the inevitable landscape of modern life. Kids needed fillings for cavities, braces for crooked teeth, and wisdom teeth extractions, and sooner or later most people lost their teeth altogether.

Dr. Price found it odd that something as essential to survival as a set of sturdy, durable teeth and healthy gums would be so poorly designed by nature and fundamentally flawed as to fail early in life. Indeed, he correctly surmised that the problems brewing in our mouths, like the ubiquitous troubles with high blood pressure, elevated cholesterol, diabetes, and clogged arteries, all were scourges that grew out of a common source—the modern diet.

In fact, cavities, tooth loss, gum disease, heart attacks and strokes are not part of the normal aging process; they are consequences of living in an alien world and consuming a diet that is foreign to our genetic identity. Dr. Price noticed a sudden deterioration in the dental health of many of his patients that seemed to coincide with the beginning of the 20th century, over 100 years ago now. He was convinced that the problem stemmed from an increasing reliance on refined white flour and sugar. He was so sure, that he quit his practice and traveled around the world, seeking out cultures where the people still lived as foragers and hunter-gatherers, as all humans once did.

Dr. Price ventured to many of the most remote and uncivilized regions of the world, documenting his findings in the book, *Nutrition and Physical Degeneration*. What he found among individuals who were still living in the wild was a remarkable absence of the degenerative diseases that plague modern populations. In these cultures, people had virtually no need for dentists or cardiologists. There was no tooth decay, no high blood pressure, and nobody was dying from heart attacks. For that matter, acne wasn't an issue either, even for the teenagers of these hunter-gatherer societies. Interestingly, this robust health was not clearly tied to just

1 special diet, but was found among groups following an extraordinary range of eating traditions. However, Dr. Price did discover that groups who subsisted on fish, seafood, wild game, vegetables, and fruits to be generally healthier than the agriculturists who ate more cereal grains, even when they were unrefined grains. Dr. Price felt that the common denominator underlying the good health of these native peoples was a traditional diet relying on fresh, whole, largely unprocessed foods from animals living in the wild and plants grown on rich soils.

One of the attributes of pure sugar or white flour that has made these foods staples of the modern diet is that they tend to keep for long periods of time. Apparently, even pests such as rodents, worms, and bacteria seem to be smarter than the modern human when it comes to dietary choices. A rat and a bacterium both instinctively understand that they cannot thrive, or even survive when eating a diet of pure calories with the nutrients stripped away, and thus foods like refined sugar and flour tend not to spoil. Yet this choice that many of us make unwittingly each day is precisely how and why most of us fall prey to the host of degenerative diseases, whether in our mouth, on our skin, or in our arteries and brain, that are commonly accepted today as a just a part of the human condition.

Healthy Mouth, Healthy Heart

When I was a 22-year-old medical student, I began to perceive that occasionally within a few hours of eating candy or a doughnut I would feel pain, redness, swelling, and maybe a bit of bleeding from 1 or 2 localized inflamed regions on my gums. An instinct told me that this was not to be ignored. I just knew somehow that the condition of my gums and teeth was not just an issue of vanity, but also a crucially important indicator about my overall state of health. Maybe it's because I noticed that people who flossed every day, like my parents and Joan's parents, had all their teeth, while those who were missing many of their teeth didn't floss. Though I must admit that, growing up 40 miles from the Canadian border, many of my friends had missing teeth because they played hockey.

Ever since then, I have followed a strict routine of flossing my teeth twice daily, on top of brushing 2 or 3 times daily, and this helps a great deal. Yet despite my diligent oral hygiene, I still noticed that my gums were very sensitive to what I ate. When I consumed things like French fries, burgers, doughnuts, cheesecake, white rice, Coke, or almost any other high-calorie, processed food that is easily digestible, I could feel the beginnings of inflammation in my gums within an hour or two. And by paying attention to these subtle clues, and modifying what I ate and drank, I figured out exactly what the ideal diet was for preventing chronic inflammation. And this as it turns out, is an essential step not just for my gums, but for achieving and maintaining optimal health and vitality for my whole body.

The accumulating science has confirmed my gut feeling, or more to the point, mouth feeling: the condition of our gums and teeth says a great deal about our overall health, especially with respect to our heart and blood vessels. Specifically, inflammation is the enemy of staying youthful and vigorous, and keeping the inflammation out of your mouth may be an important step towards preventing many of the most common, serious, chronic diseases we often develop here in modern America.

Inflammation plays an important role in the development of plaque in your blood vessels and ups your risks for any number of diseases as I've mentioned before. Periodontitis, or chronic infections in the gums, is also associated with increased inflammation in the bloodstream. Estimates vary, but somewhere between 20 to 80 percent of U.S. adults have some form of periodontal disease. Severe periodontitis, the kind that causes severe inflammation throughout the body, is seen in about 1 percent of the adult population in the United States—about 3 million people in all.

Less plaque on teeth is linked to less plaque in arteries. The recent studies about gum disease and cardiovascular health are downright frightening—infections and inflammation brewing in your gums are closely tied to the condition of your coronary arteries that supply oxygen and nutrients to your heart muscle. An impressive and startling recent trial found that by doing nothing else but aggressively clearing up the infections in the gums, researchers were able to also make the carotid arteries (these supply the brain) less inflamed and healthier as well.

Take-Home Messages

1. The health of your teeth and gums is a gauge of inflammation in your overall system.

2. Keeping your gums healthy may help to keep your arteries, heart and brain healthy.

3. FLOSS!! At least once each and every day. I jokingly tell my kids, "Flossing is optional: you only need to floss those teeth you want to keep."

4. Brush your teeth at least twice daily. Consider using a high-quality electronic toothbrush (using sound wave technology)—they tend to clean the teeth and gums more thoroughly than manual toothbrushes. Look for one that has a 2-minute timer to make sure you brush long enough during each session.

5. Strengthen your jaws and teeth by using them for what they were designed by nature to do: chew tough, whole, natural, raw foods such as nuts, crunchy vegetables (like carrots, broccoli, kale), and fruits (like apples). Strictly avoid tobacco products.

CHAPTER 10

Fast Each Night to Shine Each Day

Fasting is, without question, one of the most widely pre-scribed religious practices. A time-honored commandment of Bud-dhist, Hindu, Jewish, Muslim, and Mormon religions, these faiths teach that fasting, generally for 12 to 24 hours, purifies the mind and body, strengthens resistance, and improves concentration. An evolving scientific body of evidence confirms the fact that fasting can indeed purify the body, perhaps better than any other strategy. Studies also show that regular fasting may improve survival and reduce risks of diabetes and heart disease.

Annoyingly often, I find myself trying to discourage my patients from pursuing sham treatments such as colonic cleansing or chelation therapy in their misguided efforts to purify their body and become healthier. Perhaps they imagine that flushing out one's bowels is like hosing out a dirty garage, but in truth your body is amazingly effective at self-cleaning if you can just pause and give it a break from having to continually process calories—non-stop, 24/7.

We've been sharing in the passages above how your diet can be anti-inflammatory and reduce spikes in blood glucose and fats. Yet, the undisputed best method for preventing these spikes is to just simply not consume calories for 12 hours each night. This ensures that all the 'smoke' generated by metabolizing your last meal is cleared from your system by the next morning. This smoke billowing through your body is in the form of free radicals which in turn trigger inflammation. By simply fasting you can help to clear the inflammation, strengthen the immune system, and enhance your capabilities to heal yourself and grow stronger overnight. The old saying—"starve a fever and feed a cold" originated in

Michelangelo's era—16th century Europe. As with much cultural wisdom, it may convey some truth. Fasting for a short period of time enhances immunity especially against bacterial infections and influenza. And because the process of digestion requires substantial energy, fasting allows your body to divert more of its resources towards fighting off the infection. In contrast, a cold usually runs its course in about a week, and fasting for this length of time would be counterproductive for immunity and healing.

Fasting the Easy Way

Bill was turning 55 and was overweight. He asked if he could try a diet that involved fasting. I told him, "Each week I want you to eat 3 meals a day for 6 days, then skip a day." When he returned 6 weeks later, he had lost nearly 20 pounds. I congratulated him. "That's astounding Bill. You must be following the program closely." He nodded yes. "I'll tell you though, that seventh day nearly kills me!" I said, "So the hunger gets pretty difficult to tolerate?" Bill replied, "No, it's all that darn skippin' that nearly does me in!"

For more than 99.9 percent of our *Homo sapiens* family history we had no electric lights, refrigerators, TVs, computers, microwaves or all-night drive-thru restaurants. Shortly after we finished eating our evening meal and the daylight faded to night we retired to our beds. And we didn't eat again until sometime after the sun came up the next morning. The long night's sleep and fast provided indispensable time for healing and purifying the body and brain; leaving one feeling rested, revitalized, and recharged upon awakening the next morning.

A 12-Hour Nightly Fast Extinguishes Inflammation

You are designed to thrive and look and feel your best when you go 12 hours of each 24-hour period without consuming any calories. Why do you think it's referred to as *break-fast*? You can't break a fast if you snack right up until your midnight bedtime and then eat again upon awakening 5 hours later. The habits of staying up late and eating after dark are very recent developments in the 150,000-year sweep of human existence. So, your metabolism is hardwired to anticipate a nightly fast, which is a key time for your body to clear the inflammation from your system, and burn off belly fat to supply the energy to keep your 'furnace running' while you are sleeping.

Consume No Calories After Dinner to Burn Off Belly Fat

During daylight hours, the majority of the calories you consume are burned for fuel to power your muscles and brain. The leftover energy is converted to glycogen and stored in the liver as a source for quick fuel between meals. During the night, as you sleep and fast, your body converts any leftover glycogen back into glucose and trickles it into your bloodstream to maintain steady blood sugar levels. And when you burn through your stored glycogen, your body taps into your fat stores, and begins to melt away belly fat, which is burned for energy. So when you quit eating after your evening meal and get to bed for 8 luxurious hours of healing, age-defying, restorative beauty sleep, you will also be burning off belly fat while you snooze.

But keep in mind that it takes a few hours to deplete the day's glycogen stores. So when you snack until midnight and then gobble down a breakfast at 7:30 the next morning, your body will not have needed to melt much body fat during the night. In other words, if you limit your eating to a period of about 12 hours a day, say between about 7:30 a.m. to 7:30 p.m., you will give your body a chance to burn through all of its stored glycogen for the first half of the night, at which point it will start melting belly fat for the last several hours of the fast.

Over time, a nightly fast can transform your body composition and rejuvenate your long-term health. In a recent study published in *Cell Metabolism*, researchers found that mice fed a high-calorie diet with meals spread evenly throughout the 24-hour period became obese and diabetic; while in contrast other mice eating the same diet with the same total daily calorie intake, except concentrated in an eight-hour period, did not gain any weight and did not develop diabetes. So it appears that fasting for 12 hours might protect to some degree against many of the harmful effects of an unhealthy diet, including putting on excess belly fat and developing diabetes.

Protein and Fiber: Essential for Overnight Fasting and Losing Weight

A dinner that contains protein, fiber, and water will make it easy to get in the habit of not eating or drinking calories between the evening meal and breakfast the next morning. When you want to avoid eating for 12 hours it is essential that you are not feeling any hunger. And the recipe for long-lasting satiety is protein + fiber + hydration. Your body needs plenty of protein to rebuild tissues that are constantly breaking down. Each day you tear down about a half-pound of protein, which must be reconstructed in order to build and maintain strong muscles, sturdy bones, a healthy digestive tract, and a powerful and vigilant immune system. Eating protein will keep you full, and help you to lose excess body fat while preserving or even augmenting your valuable muscle tissue. Fiber ideally obtained from vegetables, fruits, nuts, and legumes will also help to keep you feeling full longer. Recent studies also show that a high-fiber diet is helpful at preventing cancers, especially of the digestive tract, lowering heart attack risk and improving overall life expectancy. Gulping down a 12 to 16 ounce glass of water mixed with a heaping tablespoon of sugar-free Metamucil an hour or 2 after your evening meal will help to keep you full and make it easier to fast after dinner each night.

Chapter 11

Power Up Your Brain

How to Rejuvenate Your Brain

It has been said that love is the 1 thing in life that would be most difficult to live without; though toilet paper would run a close second. I would argue that right up there at the top of that list of life's essentials is a healthy, happy, and capable brain.

As a cardiologist, I hate to admit that I consider brain health to be even more important than heart health. Worst case scenario—we can switch out your ruined heart for a transplanted heart, or even a mechanical one. But you trash your brain, and the party is over. Because you are fortunate enough to be alive in 21st century America, you can look forward to living decades longer than humans from other places and times. However, one of the major drawbacks of this increased life expectancy is that the older you get, the higher your risk for suffering from degenerative brain diseases like Alzheimer's and Parkinson's, as well as strokes. And, don't believe what one of my patients told me, "I feel like I am losing my mind, but honestly, I don't really miss it."

Fortunately, what's good for the heart is good for the brain (and bones, and kidneys, and eyes, and sex organs). Breakthrough studies indicate that your brain health is largely in your own hands. So listen up—a mind is a terrible thing to waste.

Amazingly, just 30 minutes of moderate or intense aerobic exercise can even make you smarter for the next several hours. We're not talking about the kind of smarts that come from a book;

but instead a heightened mental focus that enables quicker and more precise decision-making, enlightened creativity, and improved productivity. Research has shown that a 30-minute cardio workout can boost the raw information-processing capability of the brain, thereby improving memory and the ability to multi-task. A study of 210 workers found that on a day when they participated in an exercise program they scored 15 percent higher in their ability to meet time and output demands such that they were able to accomplish in an 8-hour day what would otherwise take them 9½ hours to do. So we aren't buying the *not enough time* excuse for being sedentary—if you need to be more resourceful, creative, focused, and energized, yet relaxed and confident, you simply cannot afford to not take time out of your day to get some exercise. Allocating 30 to 50 minutes for your daily workout may be the single most important strategy to ensure that you will thrive in your busy and demanding 21st century American life.

> "My priorities are changing. For instance, I used to exercise to keep my butt in shape, but now I exercise to keep my brain in shape."
> –Karen

Other studies show that aerobic exercise has the mental focusing effect similar to that of drugs utilized for attention deficit hyperactivity disorder (ADHD). Like a lot of problems, ADHD can be treated naturally and without prescription drugs if you will simply do what you're designed to do: move... every chance you get. Exercise will also reduce anxiety and depression; yet nearly all of the benefits of physical activity are very temporary, so we all need to exercise almost every day.

This is a no-brainer; exercise is like a wonder drug for your mind. Other studies show that exercise not only improves short-term mental functioning, but also is one of the single most important ways you can reduce your chances for developing Alzheimer's disease and other forms of dementia, as well as stroke. Exercise immediately lowers your blood pressure, blood sugar, triglycerides, and stress hormones. It makes you happier, improves self-esteem, and improves your energy levels and sleep. And the latest science shows a vigorous bout of cardio exercise will improve your ability to think clearly, deeply, and creatively. Exercise cleanses your system of the toxic effects of stress and too many calories.

Power Up Your Mind

Have a daily glass of red wine at happy hour. One 5-ounce glass of red wine a day, preferably immediately before or with your evening meal, will help to keep sugar levels from spiking after dinner, thereby preventing inflammation in the brain, and reducing the risk of Alzheimer's disease by up to 30 percent. However, remember the dangers we've already discussed about consuming more than 2 drinks a day.

Exercise every, or almost every, day. Nothing has been shown to preserve, and indeed even sharpen, brain function better than a vigorous bout of physical activity. Even 30 minutes of moderate-to-hard exercise will ramp up your ability to solve difficult problems, multi-task, and think creatively. Exercise in the morning and your improved productivity will free up extra play time at the end of the day, and give you the energy and enthusiasm to make the most of it. Astoundingly, 40 minutes or more of vigorous aerobic exercise, at least 3 times weekly for a year, was recently shown to increase the size and power of the hippocampus—the part of the brain responsible for making new memories; in the same study the hippocampus shrank in size in the group not doing regular dynamic aerobic exercise.

Omega-3 Is Brain Food

These revitalizing fats are especially important for brain health. When you eat fish or fish oil, the omega-3 fats are sopped up by the membranes that envelop every 1 of the 100 billion neurons that make the human brain—the most amazing and intelligent entity in the known universe. DHA is the specific omega-3 fat that is the most powerful for recharging the brain. Look for fish oil that is rich in DHA; you should be consuming at least 1,000 mg of DHA each day.

Hot-off-the-press research involving participants in the famous Framingham Study found that fish truly is brain food. This study, published in the journal *Neurology*, evaluated how levels of omega-3 affected both the size and function of the brain. People with higher levels of DHA did not show as much age-related brain shrinkage as those who had lower DHA levels. Even more importantly, low DHA levels were linked with poor memory and reduced ability for abstract thinking and complex reasoning. In other words, low DHA levels accelerated brain aging and brain shrinkage resulting in deterioration of thinking skills. Keep your brain plump, youthful, and razor-sharp by feeding it generous amounts of DHA from fish and/or fish oil. Similarly, brain health is another reason to ask your doctor to check your vitamin D level; most people need to supplement with vitamin D_3.

Leafy greens, like kale, and other colorful plant foods are abundant in powerful antioxidants called flavones that help to cool inflammation and fight disease. Recent studies show that the more vegetables you eat on a daily basis, the less likely you are to suffer age-related decline in mental function. Particularly the green leafy veggies such as spinach, kale, broccoli, and mixed greens are beneficial as brain-food. In one study of 3,000 age 65 or over, daily intake of 2 or more servings of leafy greens decreased the rate of decline in brain function by 40 percent.

Additionally, a diet high in antioxidants from sources such as blackberries, strawberries, raspberries, green tea, coffee, dark chocolate, and red wine can improve the function of your blood vessels by as much as 50 percent. That means healthier, less inflamed arteries, which revitalizes everything from your brain and heart to your sexual function.

Blueberries, especially wild blueberries, are a rich source of potent antioxidants called anthocyanins. These dark blue pigments in berries have been shown to enhance brain performance in humans. Recently, in a randomized controlled trial, people who consumed blueberries on a daily basis showed significant improvements in learning and memory, fewer signs of depression, and lower blood sugar levels. Try to eat a half a cup of blueberries daily.

My friend Charles is a 90-year-old genius who eats a cup of blueberries every morning while mulling over new concepts from the latest text books on theoretical mathematics and astrophysics. After reading studies describing how eating blueberries on a regular basis can lower blood pressure and maintain sharp brain function, Charles decided that blueberries, while somewhat expensive, are preferable to prescription medications... and much better tasting.

Be like Charles and try to challenge your brain by learning new things. Try learning how to speak a foreign language, or how to play a musical instrument, or how to use new computer programs and skills, or discover how to do new things with your smart phone. Go on trips and try to do your own navigating. Limit TV time. A scientific study found that people who watch more than 4 hours of TV per day were 80 percent more likely to die of cardiovascular diseases, like stroke and heart attack, during the 6-year follow-up period compared to those who spent less than 2 hours daily in front of a television. Even 2 to 4 hours of TV daily increased risk of cardiovascular death by 19 percent.

Take a low-dose aspirin (81 mg) at bedtime. This helps to protect against stroke, especially in women over age 65, and men over age 50. A recent study showed that if you take a low-dose aspirin before you go to sleep, it will lower your systolic (top) blood pressure by 5 points through the night. In contrast, when the same 81 mg aspirin is taken during the day it seems to have no effect on blood pressure.

Attitudes for a Powerful Mind at Any Age

A change of mind can mean a change of heart. Adopting the right attitudes will improve not just the quality of your life, but also the quantity.

Kindness

A gentle compassion for others radiates healing and calming effects to your own heart. Among the strongest predictors of longevity is time spent helping others and volunteering. In other words, unselfish behavior is one of the best ways to improve one's own health. The simple kindnesses you show to others will be reflected back to you, as will coldness, hostility, and selfishness.

Forgiveness

Lose the baggage. It's much easier to be light-hearted if you're not burdening your life with a load of resentments. Yogi Berra said, "I used to carry grudges until I figured out that while I was carrying the grudge, the other guy was out dancing!"

Optimism

The glass is half full, not half empty; and even if it's not—pretend it is. Sometimes rose-colored glasses can make it easier to overcome problems that might otherwise overwhelm you. Many people find that religious faith and/or spirituality can bolster their hope, gratitude, and resiliency as they deal with the ups and downs of life.

Open-mindedness

Being alive means dealing with change. The more adaptable you can stay, the longer and more vigorous your life is likely to be. Variety is the spice of life—meet new people, go new places, and do new things. Be adventurous.

Play

Had any fun lately? Make it a priority to enjoy life with the people in your world. The time and energy spent with family, friends, and pets is not an optional luxury, but instead an essential requirement for your well-being. Active play is often the best medicine, since we generally get inadequate exercise unless we make a point of engaging in vigorous activities during our free time. Physical intimacy with the love of your life on a regular basis will naturally increase your sense of bliss and well-being.

Love

Our daughter Caroline is the youngest of our 4 children. She is a charming free-spirit who often chimes up at seemingly random times to say, "I love you, Dad" or "I love you, Mom." Admittedly, she says "I love you" to everyone from her teachers to Ernie her Beta fish; but when she says that to us it always just melts our hearts. Nothing is more endearing than an expression of genuine affection. Kiss your spouse or significant other, hug your kids or grandkids and tell them how much you love them. If you want to have a friend, you have to be a friend; so make sure your pals know that they are special to you. Take the time to pet your dog or cat and nurture the plants in your yard and home. These are the behaviors and emotions that will reliably relax and rejuvenate your heart and blood vessels which will make them soft and supple like they were when you were a teen.

CHAPTER 12

Burning Off Belly Fat

Banish Belly Fat (No Crunches Required!)

There aren't many things that will do more to improve your health, or your sex appeal, than getting rid of the spare tire around your midsection. Excess belly fat, especially the kind that accumulates in and around the abdominal organs such as the liver and intestines, churns out stress hormones and inflammatory chemicals. It also predisposes to spikes in blood glucose after eating, and a host of chronic diseases. So shedding those extra inches around your waistline is not just a vanity issue; your future health and vitality are at stake.

Blood pressure tends to track very closely with your weight. If you are carrying extra weight, especially belly fat, you can be pretty sure that as your weight and waist size come down towards ideal, your blood pressure will follow. Of course it works the other way too—when you gain weight your blood pressure will generally climb. The fact that 70 percent of Americans are overweight or obese is a major reason why 9 out of 10 Americans eventually develop high blood pressure.

Here are 14 steps that will help to melt the excess belly fat off your waistline so that you can show off your sexy abs again, restoring youthful health and vigor as well.

1. Exercise daily in some way. Almost every day you need to accumulate at least 15 or 20 minutes of physical activity, and ideally up to 30 to 50 minutes of moderate or hard exercise.

2. Eat protein with each of your meals. Also, try to eat a high quality protein like whey protein or egg whites within 2 hours, before or after, of exercise.

3. Pick 2 colors with each meal—two servings or more of brightly colored veggies or fruits 3 times per day.

4. Get in the habit of having a glass of low-sodium V8® juice at breakfast.

5. Never eat until you are overfull. Eat only until you aren't hungry anymore. You may have to slow down how quickly you eat so that you can actually feel that you are no longer hungry before consuming those extra calories.

6. Drink at least 3 or 4 cups of tea, especially green tea, daily. This will bring down your blood pressure, and safely increase your metabolism to help you keep fat off your abdomen. This is particularly true if you substitute tea for diet sodas and/or calorie-rich drinks like sweetened soft drinks and sugary sports drinks. It's the antioxidants combined with the modest dose of caffeine in green tea that help burn off excess belly fat. If you can't drink enough green tea consider taking a daily tea supplement in the form of a pill. Shoot for at least 600 mg daily of the tea antioxidants.

7. If you are going to cheat and eat a decadent dessert, French fries, chips, cake, etc., follow Joan's 3-bite rule. Pick a treat, but you get only 3 bites. By the way, you only get to use the 3-bite rule 1 time per day, max.

8. Markedly cut back on starches and sugars. Eliminate essentially all white foods like white flour, white rice, potatoes, bagels, and doughnuts.

9. Drink only water (6 to 8 glasses per day), coffee, tea, and skim milk, or coconut milk. No soda pop (even diet), no artificial sweeteners, no fruit juices. Cut back on caffeine after noon. Importantly, coffee means a cup o' joe, not dressed up coffee-esque drinks that are laden with fats and sugars.

10. Sleep 7½ to 9 hours per night. This is a critical component of a belly fat-burning program. Sleep deprivation cranks up your stress hormones that make you crave junk food and then immediately deposits all those calories as fat around your waist.

11. Try to eat more healthy fats like fish oil and monounsaturated fats. Take 1,500 mg of omega-3 per day, and try to eat a handful of nuts per day. Use extra virgin olive oil for your salad dressing and cooking oil uses.

12. Take 2,000 IU of vitamin D_3 per day. Talk to your doctor to test your levels and determine if you are Vitamin D deficient, in which case you may need more.

13. Keep your alcohol intake modest, and drink mostly red wine. Why do you think it's called a beer-belly? One drink per day will reduce abdominal fat, but anything more than 2 drinks daily accumulates in and around your belly.

14. Use a soluble fiber supplement like Metamucil (sugar-free).

Fat Chance

Too many easily digestible carbohydrates increase the insulin level, stimulate your appetite, and increase fat deposition especially in the abdominal area. Too much stress elevates cortisol, which compels you to eat constantly and also deposits fat around your belly. Sedentary living blunts growth hormone production, whereas vigorous physical exercise is the best way to increase adult growth hormone level, which gives a powerful boost to energy, vitality, and a youthful appearance. Weight lifting will increase your testosterone levels, making it easier to build muscle. Realigning your hormone profile by following the recommendations of the Forever Young program also provides many other anti-aging benefits such as an improved complexion, more lean muscle, less male pattern balding, stronger bones and teeth, improved sex drive, better sleep, fewer nighttime awakenings to empty your bladder, more energy, better memory, and a happy focused state of mind.

Americans are getting heftier and heftier. The proportion of overweight or obese children, ages 6 to 11, doubled between 1980 and 2000, and tripled among adolescents ages 12 to 17. Even older Americans are becoming plump; today 7 out of 10 people between ages 55 and 74 are overweight, which is about twice the prevalence 30 years ago. A study of 73,000 adults published in the *American Journal of Preventive Medicine* showed that having excess body fat significantly increased risk for a wide range of problems, including coronary disease, heart failure, blood clots in the veins, high blood pressure, depression, sleep disorders, indigestion, erectile dysfunction, arthritis, hip and knee replacements, asthma, and diabetes.

The journal *The Lancet* published a paper that found that obesity accelerates aging by destroying telomeres—remember, these are the caps on the ends of chromosomes that prevent the DNA from fraying. In this study of 1,222 British women, the telomere shortening indicated that obesity caused about 8.8 years of accelerated aging as compared to the lean women. These increased health problems and premature aging are largely due to disturbances in hormonal and chemical balances in the body and brain often seen in overweight and obese individuals. Adding insult to injury, obesity also unfairly affects job salary. Sociologist Dalton Conley, PhD, found that in women, but not men, every 10 percent increase in weight correlated with a 6 percent decrease in income. So it's very important that you get your eating and lifestyle under control and get back to a healthy weight range.

Simply measuring the waist size is the easiest and most practical marker of obesity since the most dangerous and detrimental fat is that which is deposited inside your abdominal cavity. By the way, your belt size is not always an accurate indicator of your waist circumference, especially in men who typically wear their belt somewhere south of their true waist. As a rule of thumb, the waist is the part of the body that is the first to enter a room as you walk through the doorway. Measure your waist about 1 inch above your belly button (or about half way between your belly button and the lower edge of your rib cage on your side). Ideal waist circumference is less than half your height in inches. For example, a 6 foot man should have a waist circumference less that 36 inches; a 5′6″ woman's waist should be less than 33 inches. A waist circumference of over 35 inches for a woman or over 40 inches for a man is a serious health warning sign because excessive fat around the midsection is usually associated with inflammation of the blood vessels and increased risk of cardiovascular disease, diabetes, and high blood pressure.

Take Your Health into Your Own Hands

The last person without a college education to occupy the Oval Office of the White House was our home town hero, here in Kansas City, President Harry Truman. He lived to almost 90 years of age and for all but the last few months, conveyed the picture of hale and hearty good health. His complexion glowed, he stood with his shoulders back and he carried himself with optimism, confidence, and ease. He also maintained a happy disposition while coping with the ominous and overwhelming burdens as the American Commander-in-Chief during one of the most critical junctures in modern history—1944 through 1952.

When asked about his secret to good health he replied, "I eat no bread except for an occasional small piece of toast at breakfast, no butter, no sugar, and no sweets. Usually I have fruit, 1 egg, 1 strip of bacon, and a half-glass of skimmed milk for breakfast. I eat fish, spinach, and another nonfattening vegetable for lunch, with fruit for dessert. For dinner I have a cup of fresh fruit, steak, a couple of non-fattening vegetables and an ice orange, pineapple, or raspberry. So, I maintain my waist line and can wear suits bought in 1935!"

Sixty years ago Harry Truman's daily routine included 8 servings of fresh vegetables and fruits, 3 servings of protein, and virtually no added sugars, with minimal grains and refined foods. He also walked 2 miles each morning at a brisk pace, "As if I had somewhere important to be," as Harry described it. He also did some sit-ups and other calisthenics, and then often received a massage. Harry made a habit of drinking about 1 shot of whiskey each day. He put his family first, loved to play the piano, and had an irrepressible sense of humor.

How was it that this farm boy who graduated from high school in Independence, Missouri, over 100 years ago managed to figure out, apparently on his own, the ideal diet and lifestyle for fostering health, resilience, happiness, and longevity? The same way Joan's mother, Kathleen, personally discovered the secrets to health and longevity some 6 decades ago. When Kathleen was a fit and active 31-year-old administrative assistant working for the U.S. Navy in Hawaii in 1944, a doctor, on the basis of an erroneous blood glucose test, told her she had diabetes. In fact, she was not diabetic at the time, and never was; but the health-scare roused this already conscientious young woman into becoming a zealot about her diet. She voraciously read everything about healthy eating that she could find. Joan remembers her mother sitting cross-legged on her bed with books, magazines, and newspaper articles strewn all around her, intent on deciphering the truth about nutrition, and harnessing the science that would give her the personal power to stay healthy and strong. She embraced a diet of steamed vegetables, salads of leafy greens (spinach especially) mixed with tomatoes and carrots and dressed with olive oil and vinegar, fresh colorful fruits, fish, modest servings of lean meats, nuts, water, tea, and coffee with a moderate daily alcohol use. Kathleen, until her death at 99, still enjoyed life, lived independently in her own home, ran her successful real estate business, and exercised every day. She was still fascinated by the latest science on nutrition, and we often found her reading at her living room table which was always strewn with health and wellness literature.

Like Harry and Kathleen, if you use your intuition and pay close attention to what makes you thrive and feel fully alive, you will instinctively come to understand how to eat, play, rest, and live. When you consume a diet of natural unprocessed foods, and make a point to, on a daily basis, get exercise, fresh air, and plenty of rest, you feel better immediately; you won't need to live to 90 or 100 to know for sure that this is the path to vitality and longevity. Ironically, while many so-called experts are still arguing about these issues, enlightened individuals have intuitively understood for centuries the essence of what constitutes an ideal diet and lifestyle. Yet the average American is so confused by conflicting messages about nutrition, the marketing of fast food/ junk food, and their harried lifestyle that he or she doesn't know what to believe or how to eat, and thus defaults back to the auto-destructive standard American diet and lifestyle. However, if you reconnect with your body and tune in to how you feel when you follow our plan for living and eating you will discover in only a few days that the concepts can be felt first hand and instinctively understood.

"I know the price of success: dedication, hard work, and an unremitting devotion to the things you want to see happen."
–Frank Lloyd Wright

Your life is defined by your choices. Make up your mind to take control of your own destiny. Investing the time and effort necessary to regain optimum health should be among your top day-to-day priorities. Commit yourself to continual self-improvement, and confidently follow your dreams to develop the life that you have imagined.

Our Biggest Loser

When I first met Jim Slayton 9 years ago, he tipped the scales at 401 pounds. This good-natured, retired over-the-road trucker suffered from a long list of health problems including a very weak heart muscle—a disease known as cardiomyopathy. He had several other serious conditions including atrial fibrillation (an irregular heartbeat), a leaking heart valve, sleep apnea, diabetes, arthritis, high cholesterol, high blood pressure, and gout. "I couldn't walk 30 feet without being out of breath, and exhausted," Jim said. "I felt pretty bad."

To be honest, as his cardiologist, I was very worried that if he was not able to turn things around soon, Jim's survival would be in jeopardy. An emergency trip to the Mid-America Heart Institute of St. Luke's Hospital served as a wake-up call Jim will never forget. "I had been on the tractor out mowing the pasture, and when I came inside the house, I passed out," he said. When he arrived at the hospital, the gurney collapsed under his weight, and in the cardiac catheterization lab, the doctors were concerned that he might be too heavy for the treatment table.

"That was pretty embarrassing," Jim said. "I made up my mind I needed to do something about my weight, right then and there." When he returned home, Jim decided his weight loss plan would include 2 important components of a healthy lifestyle— walking and a balanced diet.

At first, walking wasn't easy for Jim, but he started slowly and gradually built up his endurance. "I started by walking around the house twice a day," Jim said. Six months later, he was walking 2 miles a day. Today, he walks 5 to 6 miles each day, logging nearly 2,400 miles last year alone. "When the weather is reasonable, I walk on the blacktop road near my home for about 2 hours. When it's bad, I walk for the same amount of time around the edge of my basement. I'm not crazy about treadmills."

Watching his diet was tough too. Jim said. "I'm a food-a-holic. I think I was born heavy. I could eat all the time. The trick to losing weight and keeping it off is to stay away from unhealthy foods, and eat a balanced diet, including lots of fruits and vegetables. We don't overeat; and now my wife Sandy and I are careful about not bringing home junk food."

One year after Jim's wake-up call, he had lost 150 pounds. Over the next year he shed another 65 pounds to reach his goal of 185 pounds; 216 pounds lighter than when he started his new life. And since then, he's kept the weight off by diligently sticking to his diet and exercise plan. From a medical standpoint, Jim's multitude of life-threatening diseases have all melted away, along with his excess fat tissue.

Don't believe those advertisements that promise that you will lose 10 pounds in 48 hours—the only way to do that is to come down with the stomach flu or food poisoning! Jim's recipe for losing weight is exactly what we advise: daily exercise and our Forever Young Diet. Jim said he knew he needed to lose weight, he just didn't realize how much better he would feel when he did. "Losing weight wasn't easy, but it has a lot of benefits," Jim said. "All of my health problems are gone. My clothes are less expensive and I enjoy life more, socializing with friends, fishing, and going to auctions and antique malls. Walking daily and eating healthy have given me my life back."

CHAPTER 13

Alcohol: The Razor-Sharp Double-Edged Sword

"It has long been recognized that the problems with alcohol relate not to the use of bad things,
but to the abuse of a good thing."
–Abraham Lincoln

Paradoxically, alcohol is one of the most common causes of premature death, yet it can also be a habit that helps to confer longevity and well-being. Alcohol is the proverbial double-edged sword; and no other health factor is capable of cutting so deeply in either direction depending upon how it is used. Science shows that light to moderate drinking done on a daily basis improves cardiovascular health and substantially reduces risk of death. On the other hand, excessive alcohol intake and/or binge drinking is toxic to the heart and overall health, and is the third leading cause of premature death among Americans.

Missouri's own Harry Truman, as I shared earlier, one of the healthiest and longest-lived of the American presidents, started off each day, before his morning walk, with 1 shot of bourbon whiskey. Now, I am not suggesting that you start your day with an 'eye opener,' but it is quite likely that his routine of consuming just 1 or 2 alcoholic beverages daily (he often enjoyed a glass of wine with his evening meal) contributed to his exceptional vigor and longevity. The developing scientific consensus indicates that the specific alcoholic beverage you drink is less important than the quantity of alcohol and the pattern of intake. Having 1 drink daily (or up to 2 drinks daily for men) appears to be the ideal drinking pattern for improving cardiovascular health. Some studies suggest that wine, particularly red wine, might be the healthiest form of alcohol; but most studies show almost as much protection from any alcoholic beverage.

It is the small amount of alcohol (ethanol) itself, rather than any other specific component of the wine, beer, or spirits, that is the major factor in bestowing health benefits. A small daily dose of alcohol, ideally about 7 to 13 grams (which is about the amount of alcohol in ½ to 1 drink), reduces fats and sugar in the bloodstream and decreases inflammation, but only temporarily—for about 12 to 24 hours. This is probably why drinking a small amount 5 to 7 days a week is more heart-healthy than just occasional alcohol use. So alcohol intake, like exercise, is best done daily and in moderation. From a health standpoint, a drink immediately before or during your evening meal is ideal. Still, try to avoid drinking within 3 or 4 hours of your bedtime, since alcohol can disturb your deep, restorative sleep and/or worsen sleep apnea.

In the *American Journal of Cardiology* I and my colleagues published a study of 800 U.S. cardiovascular physicians that showed about 3 out of 4 drank alcohol regularly, with nearly half of those consuming 1 or 2 drinks a day; suggesting that American cardiologists personally recognize the potential health benefits of light to moderate regular alcohol intake.

Light to moderate drinking lowers risk of heart attack and cardiac death by approximately 30 to 35 percent, which for example, is about as much cardiovascular risk reduction as we see with the powerful statin cholesterol drugs. A recent study showed that people who were already following all of the 4 major healthy lifestyle behaviors (not smoking, maintaining a healthy weight, exercising 30 minutes a day, and eating a healthy diet) still had a

45 percent lower risk of heart attack if they were drinking a light to moderate alcohol on a regular basis. Other studies show that consuming 1 or 2 drinks daily reduces the risk of stroke, congestive heart failure, high blood pressure, and even Alzheimer's disease; but again, heavier alcohol intake progressively increases the risk for each of these problems.

A small to moderate dose of alcohol also reduces the risk of diabetes by about 30 percent. Evidence indicates that light to moderate drinking might even be good for weight control, especially for reducing belly fat. People who have 1 or 2 drinks a day seem to have less abdominal obesity than do non-drinkers, but those who consume more than 2 drinks a day have—you guessed it—a larger beer-belly, which expands in proportion to the amount of alcohol consumed.

Although Mark Twain once quipped, "Everything in moderation, including moderation," in fact even occasional immoderate drinking is bad for your health. Regular drinking is a slippery slope that many individuals cannot safely navigate; and let's be clear, getting drunk on Saturday night is not heart healthy. Binge drinking, defined as more than 5 drinks per drinking day, increases the risk of heart attack and other problems like motor vehicle accidents, stroke, dangerous heart rhythms, sudden death, suicide, cancer, liver disease, and death from all causes. Some studies suggest that alcohol abuse and binge drinking are on the rise, and alcohol abuse is currently the third largest preventable cause of death, killing more than 100,000 Americans each year.

A large study of women showed that even small doses of alcohol, about 3 to 6 drinks per week can increase risk of cancer by about 15 percent compared to women who drink no alcohol. More importantly, at higher intakes the risk of cancer rises proportionately, with the cancer risk rising about 10 percent for every drink per day consumed. So women who drink large amounts of alcohol have markedly increased risks for developing cancer. If you have personal or family history that suggests you are at high risk of cancer, it might be best to avoid alcohol entirely.

I asked Helen, one of my patients, if she drank alcohol and she replied, "Sure. I drink wine in the evening." When I asked her how much she told me, "One." So I pressed her further, "How many ounces would that be, Helen?" She told me, "I'm not sure how many ounces there are in 1 box of wine."

For the record, 1 drink is considered to be 12 ounces of beer, 5 ounces of wine, or 1.5 ounces of 80-proof spirits. If you drink alcohol responsibly, you can take heart in the knowledge that it is good for your health. However, if in the past you have had problems with abuse of alcohol or other substances, or if you smoke or have a history of depression, or have moral or religious objections to alcohol use, or have chronic health issues like severe liver disease that make alcohol use more dangerous, you should avoid alcohol use altogether. As always, it is a good idea to discuss issues or questions about alcohol with your physician when you come in for your visit.

Snuggle into the Safe Mid-Zone of Life's U-Curves

It's the Goldilocks rule of biology: not too hot, not too cold. Life tends to thrive best in average or moderate conditions—extremes are generally not conducive to health or longevity. Your life is likely to be happier, healthier, and longer if you remember that just because a little is good, more is not necessarily better; indeed oftentimes less is more. In the science of medicine, we call this phenomenon the U-shaped curve.

It amazes me how often this truism—all things in moderation—turns out to be the best advice for people looking to follow an ideally healthy lifestyle. It's out there on the edges of that

U-curve where the dangers lurk. So think of that middle zone on the bottom of the U as a platform upon which to build a nest that will keep you safe and healthy during your life.

Below are a few examples of the ubiquitous U-curves in health and medicine:

Alcohol

Hermann Smith-Johannson, a Norwegian-Canadian who was an avid cross-country skier until shortly before his death at age 103 said, "The secret to a long life is to stay busy, get plenty of exercise and don't drink too much. Then again, don't drink too little." Indeed, 1 drink a day will do everything from improve life expectancy, to lower risks for heart attack, diabetes, and dementia. However, at intakes of more than 1 drink daily for a woman or 2 drinks daily for a man, your risks increase for cancer, atrial fibrillation, heart failure, high blood pressure, and premature death (just to name a few).

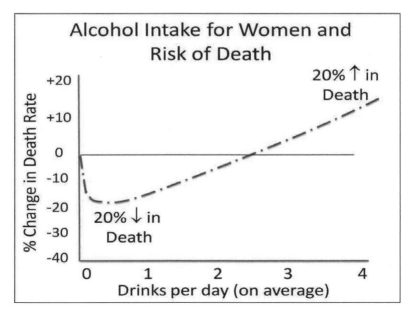

Source: O'Keefe, et al, *JACC* 2007;50:1009-1014

Blood Pressure

Ideally, your top blood pressure number (the systolic reading) should usually run between 100 and 140. You probably know that high blood pressure can kill you and cause stroke, heart attack, and heart failure. But blood pressure that's too low can make you feel light-headed, weak, and tired, cause you to pass out, and rarely, can even cause heart attacks and strokes. The bottom blood pressure number (diastolic reading) is far less important than the top.

Blood Sugar

Shoot for fasting blood glucose between 75 and 100. A reading of 100 or higher is pre-diabetes, and above 125 is diabetes. Yet, blood sugar that's too low is also problematic, and will make you feel weak and confused, and may even predispose you to serious cardiac problems.

Exercise

Vigorous exercise is like a miracle for your health—and more is better up to about 50 minutes a day. Efforts beyond that might help you burn more calories or get in shape for ultra-endurance races, but it is a point of diminishing returns when it comes to your overall health and life expectancy. Particularly after age 50, excessive and intense endurance exercise can inflict serious damage to your cardiovascular health. In contrast, a dip in the pool does wonders for an aging body. A new study from the *American Journal of Cardiology* found that swimming lowered blood pressure and made arteries more soft, supple, and responsive. And if you have issues with sore joints and muscles, swimming is a great way to exercise vigorously without stressing your joints.

Weight

Towards the end of her office visit I mentioned to Deborah that I was happy with everything except for her weight and fitness level. When I said, "You just need to get back in shape," she replied, "Hey, round is a shape, right?" When it comes to the effect of your weight on your health and longevity, being too fat isn't good, but neither is being too thin. Yet, by far the most important number to focus on is measured in inches not pounds. Shoot for a waist size that is not more than half your height in inches. See our comments on this topic earlier in Chapter 12 for more details. The significance of weight falls away if you can trim your tummy fat back to your youthful shape.

Sleep

Ideally, you should be sleeping 7½ to 9 hours each 24-hour cycle. People who chronically sleep less than 6.5 hours nightly or more than 9 hours generally aren't as healthy as the more moderate sleepers.

Stress

Unless you have lived your life in a beer commercial, you probably, at some point, have felt the corrosive effects of too much stress, which can take the fun out of life and destroy your health and well-being. While excessive stress, or distress, causes anxiety and depression, good stress (or eustress) can challenge us to overcome obstacles, learn something new, or exercise robustly, and in the process grow stronger and more resilient and find fulfillment. Just as muscles and bones grow atrophied, weak, and sickly when they are relieved of all physical demands, a human being thrives best when he or she has something to push against, goals to achieve, expectations to live up to, and causes for which to fight. Many people dream of retirement thinking that by avoiding all their work-related stress they will be happy, only to see their health and vitality diminish when they no longer have any work stress.

Vitamins and Hormones

Your body will function best when your levels of essential nutrients and important hormones are in the ideal moderate ranges: not too low, but not too high either. We will explore this topic in more detail in the next chapter.

"Perhaps too much of anything is as bad as too little."
–Edna Ferber

CHAPTER 14

The Truth About Vitamins

Essential Nutrients

Essential nutrients are so deemed because we need to get just enough of these substances on a regular basis in order to be strong and healthy. But just because a little is good, doesn't necessary mean that a lot is better. Indeed, in most of the largest and best done trials, mega-dose vitamins tend to not be beneficial to health and longevity, and in some instances, may even cause harm. But here's a key point to understand: supplementing with an essential nutrient to increase an already normal level to a super-normal (very high) level generally doesn't provide health benefits. On the other hand, taking a supplement to bring an abnormally low level of an essential nutrient into a normal range typically provides wide-ranging and powerful benefits to health and longevity.

Between the 12th and the 17th centuries, strapping young sailors with robust health boarded ships in London, Venice, or Lisbon bound for the New World, or the Far East. After a few weeks on the high seas, subsisting on salted meat, biscuits, and rum, the previously healthy men started to grow weak and sickly. While at sea with no access to fruits or vegetables for months, they developed full-blown scurvy due to severe vitamin C deficiency, which killed up to half of the sailors on very long sea voyages. Then in 1750, James Lind, a Scottish doctor in the Royal British Navy, discovered that if he squeezed lime juice (hence the nickname Limey for an Englishman) on the men's rations, they dramatically and quickly regained their hearty good health. In contrast, several modern studies have randomized thousands of healthy people to high dose vitamin C or placebo and have shown no benefits whatsoever. To the sailors with scurvy, vitamin C was a miraculous, life-saving cure; but vitamin C provided no demonstrable benefit for those with normal vitamin C levels at baseline. The important point: try to get nearly virtually all of your nutrients from eating natural whole foods; for those few essential nutrients for which your diet may be inadequate, take a supplement to bring those levels into the normal ranges.

Omega-3 and Vitamin D: The Dynamic Duo

And what essential nutrients are most likely to be lacking in the average 21st century Americans? Omega-3 fats and vitamin D. No coincidence then that among the nutrients tested in large randomized trials, omega-3 and vitamin D are the ones that have shown the most promise for providing wide-ranging health benefits. We recommend that you get at least 1,500 mg daily of DHA and EPA (the 2 most important omega-3 fats), and at least 2,000 IU daily of vitamin D_3. Keep in mind that most people need more than 2,000 IU of vitamin D_3 to keep their levels of 25-hydroxy vitamin D in the ideal range between about 30 and 60 ng/ml; and we suggest that you have your vitamin D levels measured so as to more precisely dose your vitamin D supplementation. If you frequently consume fatty fish like salmon, and are in tropical sun a great deal, you may not need either omega-3 or vitamin D supplements.

The latest vitamin to flame out in a large randomized trial was vitamin E. We have suspected for some time that high dose (400 to 1,000 IU) of vitamin E might slightly increase risk for potentially life-threatening bleeding into the brain. Now a large trial found a small, but statistically significant, increased risk of prostate cancer in men who took a 400 IU vitamin E for 7 years. The recommended minimum intake of vitamin E is only 33 IU, and that is best obtained through eating foods such as nuts, extra virgin olive oil, and avocados. Although a separate supplement of vitamin E is not a good idea, the modest vitamin E doses, about 75 IU or less that are found in multivitamins, appear to be harmless and might even provide some benefits for individuals who are not eating an ideal diet.

Folic acid is another nutrient that seemed to have compelling logic for improving cardiovascular health, but subsequent randomized trials showed no benefits. For example, the Norwegian Vitamin Trial found that a daily supplement containing 800 mcg folic acid (the synthetic form of folate used in vitamins) slightly increased the risk of having a heart attack or stroke among 3,749 people during a 3.5 year follow-up period after an initial heart attack. In contrast, people with the highest intake of folate (found in foods like avocados and leafy greens) from their diet have lower risks of developing Alzheimer's disease and heart disease. Bottom line: get your folic acid from your diet, but do not take a folic acid supplement.

Searching the World Over for the Best Omega-3

Over a century ago my great grandfather, as a newborn baby, emigrated with his family from the fjord region of Norway to northern Minnesota. One of my life's ambitions had been to get over to that part of Norway to do some sea kayaking in the fjords. About 2 years ago, I, along with my 2 sons Jimmy and Evan, my good friend Corey, and my brother Kevin, landed in a small airport in northern Norway. After traveling by car along winding narrow roads through thickly-forested, glacier-covered mountains, we arrived at Hotel Union on Geiranger fjord late one night. At the breakfast buffet the next morning I was curious to find a tray full of small plastic cups, each filled with a shot of fish oil + vitamin D.

For centuries, the hardy people living in Norway have consumed fish and/or fish oil as part of their daily routine. According to their cultural wisdom, handed down from generation to generation, it was essential to take cod liver oil daily during all months that contained an "R" in their name. For reasons unbeknownst to them, cod liver oil seemed to grant benefits to one's well-being including a sharp mind and happy mood, robust cardiovascular health, and a strong immune system. Especially in the long, cold, overcast, winter with very little sunlight, a daily intake of cod liver oil was considered vital for good health. Modern science is just now confirming the ingenuity of that folk medicine tradition.

My scientific motive behind this trip was to meet Leif Gjendemsjo in Ålesund, Norway, to discuss the new science and technology he was pioneering to produce higher purity, better-tasting omega-3 from fish oil. Leif grew up in a family of commercial fisherman. By the time he was 17 years old he had begun to explore how to get more value and benefit out of the fish beyond just selling it locally for food. In the 30 years since then, Leif, with a team of very bright scientists and engineers, has been pushing the frontiers in the field of omega-3 production and purification. I have regularly visited him and his omega-3 production facility situated on an island of stunning natural beauty surrounded by the pristine waters in the North Sea.

Fascinating data published in the *Journal of the American Medical Association*, by Nobel Prize winner Elizabeth Blackburn and her colleagues, showed that people with high blood levels of omega-3 fats tend to age more slowly than those with lower blood levels. By slowing telomere shortening, omega-3 fats appear to increase life expectancy. Indeed, omega-3 intake is associated with improved longevity and reduced risks for many of the common degenerative conditions of aging, such as Alzheimer's disease, heart disease, and macular degeneration. We strongly suggest that you can avoid the nasty-tasting, less purified fish oils and instead opt for a highly concentrated, mercury-free and purified, pleasant-tasting product.

Omega-3 to Keep You Young and Sexy

A recent study from scientists at Gettysburg College in Pennsylvania reported that by taking 4,000 mg of concentrated fish oil per day you can reduce your excess body fat while at the same time increasing muscle mass. The researchers found that the high dose omega-3 lowered levels of the stress hormone cortisol, and also reduced inflammation. Other recent studies show that people who are exercising regularly can be much more successful in losing excess weight if they add high dose omega-3 to their daily regimen.

A high intake of omega-3 helps to build and maintain strong bones too. So if you are not taking a highly purified and concentrated fish oil supplement, you could be missing an opportunity to burn of some of that unsightly and unhealthy belly fat, while at the same time gaining some health-promoting and sexy-looking muscle tissue. If building strong muscles and bones and burning off excess belly fat are key steps in your quest to stay youthful, vigorous, and sexy—harness the power of omega-3 to accomplish your goals.

Lifelong Strong Bones and Soft Supple Arteries

I personally make it a point to avoid any and all unnecessary exposure to ionizing radiation (x-rays or gamma rays from medical tests like routine dental x-rays, CT scans, nuclear tests, etc.), and take the same approach for my family and patients. Even so, many individuals on rare occasions need a CT scan, which is a powerful and essential diagnostic tool in modern medicine. The CardioScan, for example, is a CT scan using a relatively small dose of x-rays focused on the heart, looking for calcium in the coronary arteries—unmistakable evidence of atherosclerotic plaques. I read hundreds of these scans per week, and often point out to my medical students, and doctors in training that many people by middle age or older end up accumulating calcium in their arteries at the same time the calcium is being leached out of their bones. It is not uncommon to see people with more calcium in their coronary arteries than their backbones. This is a very ominous sign of old age and disease: bony arteries and soft bones. When we are young and strong our bones are rock solid and our arteries are soft and supple. Calcium is an important nutrient, but you want it in your bones and teeth—where it essential for musculoskeletal integrity, strength, and resiliency; not in our arteries—where it predisposes to heart attacks and strokes.

Next to multivitamins, calcium pills are the most commonly consumed daily over-the-counter supplement. Unfortunately, recent studies suggest that calcium supplements might increase risk of heart attack, probably by accelerating calcified plaque build-up in the coronary arteries. On the other hand, meeting your calcium requirement by getting it from your food and beverages appears to be perfectly safe, both for your bones and your heart. The traditional focus in nutrition on supplementation of single isolated nutrients may be especially misguided in the case of calcium. A diet supplemented with calcium, as a mono-nutrient pill, is not ideal for promoting bone health and may instead accelerate arterial plaque calcification and increase cardiovascular risk. A diet rich in plants such as leafy greens, colorful vegetables, and fruits will make your system less acidic, which is conducive for building and maintaining strong bones. However, plants are relatively poor sources of calcium compared to animal sources. Non-fat or low-fat dairy products such as skim milk, Greek yogurt, and kefir are excellent sources of calcium, but many adults do not tolerate dairy due to lactase deficiency or milk allergies.

Strong Bones Are Essential for Longevity

Kathleen, Joan's mother, lived for nearly 99 years in almost perfect health; she might still be alive today if her bones had not failed her. Unbeknownst to Kathleen, she was developing weak bones in middle age due to inadequate intake of calcium and vitamin D and no weight lifting. Starting about age 90 she had several falls which caused compression fractures in her spine and left her badly stooped over with constant back and neck pains. Eventually the osteoporosis ruined her health and took her life. When she fell at age 98 and broke her hip, she never recovered and died a few weeks later.

Joan is especially vigilant about building strong bones after witnessing the devastation that osteoporosis wrought upon her mother. About 2 out of 3 Americans do not meet the Recommended Daily Allowance (RDA) for calcium, which partly explains why osteoporosis or osteopenia (inadequate bone density) affects the majority of post-menopausal women and is increasingly common in men. Joan and I agree that an adequate intake of calcium, about 1,000 mg daily, is very important for building and maintaining strong bones. This is especially important today, because if you are being conscientious about your health, like Kathleen was, your chances of living into your 80s and 90s are very good; which means that you will need a sturdy and durable skeleton. Calcium supplements, however, are not a good idea, as they may increase risk of heart attack. Joan drinks 1 or 2 glasses of skim milk daily. Since I am lactose intolerant I don't drink cow's milk, but I usually have 1 serving daily of plain unsweetened Greek yogurt (I take 2 lactase tablets before I eat my yogurt). I also drink 1 or 2 glasses of unsweetened coconut milk daily. High intake of dairy, over 2 servings daily, has been linked to higher risks for prostate cancer and Parkinson's disease, and because I have an uncle who has had both of those problems I limit my dairy to 1 or less serving daily.

Adult human hunter-gatherers for millennia acquired most of their calcium by consuming animal bones, where it is found in a matrix of bone-building nutrients including magnesium, phosphorus, and protein. I know—eating bones during your meals is currently inconvenient and socially impolite, yet it may be a key to strong bones and soft, supple arteries. Make stews using bones, letting them slow cook for hours. And if you like sardines, look for those with the skin and bones intact, packed in water with no added salt. Consuming plenty of high-quality protein like egg whites, whey protein, lean red meat and fish, when combined with adequate calcium and magnesium intake and regular strength training (like weight lifting), is a sure-fire recipe for strong bones that will hold up for a century.

Strategies for lifelong soft, supple arteries and resilient and strong bones include the following steps:

1. Exercise daily. Yes, this is another reason to exercise. Make sure you are doing some strength training, or carrying heavy objects frequently. I have always been skinny, which is a risk factor for osteopenia and osteoporosis, so I look for opportunities to bear weight to keep my frame sturdy. If you happen to see me in the airport, I will have a backpack on my shoulders, and will be carrying (rather than rolling) a suitcase, while I climb the stairs rather than ride up escalator. By nature, we are designed to be carrying heavy things our whole lives; we need these kind of physical stresses to be optimally tough and hardy. Tote your own groceries from the store to the car. Nurture plants in your yard; gardening presents many opportunities to improve your musculoskeletal toughness and resilience via lifting heavy objects, sunlight exposure, bending and stretching. Do weight lifting 2 or 3 times weekly.

2. Keep your vitamin D levels high. It is important to maintain normal vitamin D levels from sun exposure and/or intake of oral vitamin D_3. Most people need to take at least 2,000 IU of vitamin D_3 daily. Many people need up to 6,000 IU daily to keep their vitamin D levels in the optimal range of 30 to 60 ng/ml. Make sure you have your vitamin D levels tested if you are taking more than 3,000 IU or more of vitamin D daily.

3. Consume calcium from foods and beverages. We recommend that adults about 1,000 mg of calcium daily. If you are not

lactose intolerant, you can consume up to 2 servings of low-fat or fat-free dairy daily. If you are lactose intolerant, consider taking lactase pills or drink Lactaid milk (which has lactase mixed into it already). Unsweetened coconut milk from Trader Joe's is my favorite calcium rich beverage (about 300 mg per 8 ounce glass). Calcium from animal sources, such as non-fat or low-fat dairy and sardines with the bones and skin intact, are easily absorbed. Lifelong, robust, resilient skeletal health is dependent upon eating adequate amounts of calcium, but avoid taking a calcium supplement.

4. <u>Maintain proper acid-base balance</u>. You can do this by avoiding grains and refined carbs (any processed or refined grain products or those containing added sugar or high-fructose corn syrup). Carbonated sodas like colas will also acidify your system and erode your bones. Sparkling water (flavored or plain) is perfectly healthy, just be sure to choose unsweetened varieties. Eat at least 2 colors for each of your 3 meals per day. Along with 1 serving per meal of lean fresh protein.

5. <u>Do not smoke</u>. I don't think I need to explain this one.

6. <u>Use toothpaste with fluoride and drink tea</u> (which is fluoride-rich).

7. <u>Make sure you get enough vitamin K</u>. Vitamin K_2 is especially helpful for maintaining strong bones. This form of vitamin K is hard to get from diet, so it is best to supplement with about 1–5 mg per day of vitamin K_2.

8. <u>Develop good posture</u>. On a daily basis, work on maintaining ideal posture.

Magnesium: the Wonder Mineral

Magnesium is an essential mineral that supports healthy heart and brain function, lowers blood pressure and blood sugar, and contributes to the construction of strong bones. Unfortunately, the modern diet that is high in processed food is low in magnesium, leaving about 2-thirds of American adults with blood levels of magnesium that are less than ideal.

Magnesium is an essential co-factor for many of the metabolic reactions that generate and burn energy, and thus it stands to reason that low magnesium blood levels are implicated in obesity and diabetes. New studies indicate that magnesium deficiency, among other adverse effects, causes premature aging at the genetic level, by accelerating shortening of the telomere (the caps at the end of your chromosomes that prevent the DNA from unraveling). Indeed, chronic magnesium deficiency increases the risk for age-related chronic degenerative and inflammatory conditions such as cardiovascular disease, high blood pressure, osteoporosis, dementia, and some cancers.

Conventional wisdom has suggested that the ideal ratio of mineral intake calls for 2 parts calcium for every 1 part magnesium. However, our prehistoric hunter-gatherer ancestors ate a diet that had a calcium/magnesium ratio of approximately one-to-one, with a much higher intake of magnesium compared to modern diets. Moreover, magnesium promotes concurrent calcium absorption from a meal. In contrast, excess calcium intake interferes with magnesium uptake.

An accumulating body of scientific evidence suggests that increasing intake of magnesium in the form of diet and/or supplements may provide a host of health benefits, including reduced risks for diabetes, osteoporosis, Alzheimer's disease, and coronary heart disease. A study in the March 2011 issue of the journal *Diabetes, Obesity and Metabolism* reported that 345 mg of magnesium in the form of a pill supplement significantly lowered both blood sugar and blood pressure in a group of pre-diabetic individuals.

A person who is deficient in magnesium is much more likely to develop dangerous heart rhythms. A recent study found that among 14,000 people, low magnesium blood levels significantly increased risk of sudden cardiac arrest. Harvard researchers evaluating data from the Nurses' Health Study concluded that women with higher magnesium levels were about 50 percent less likely to have suffered sudden cardiac arrest during long-term follow-up.

Best Dietary Sources of Magnesium

The recommended daily allowance of magnesium is 320 mg for women and 420 mg for men. Because of the far-reaching and significant health benefits associated with this mineral, I personally take a daily supplement of 300 mg of magnesium. I also eat a diet rich in magnesium. Top food sources of magnesium are:

- Almonds or cashews   235 mg per 3 oz.

- Spinach   160 mg per 1 cup, cooked

- King salmon   122 mg per 3 oz., cooked

- Halibut   100 mg per 3 oz., cooked

- Black beans   120 mg per 1 cup, cooked

- Egg whites   98 mg per 2 egg whites

- Skim or 1% milk   50 mg per 8 fluid oz.

Other high-magnesium food sources include leafy green vegetables, beans, chicken, and red meat. Bottom line: make sure your diet is loaded with foods that are high in magnesium, and you may even want to consider a daily supplement of 250 to 400 mg of magnesium.

Naked at Noon—The Power of Vitamin D

Unless you are lying naked at midday without sunscreen on your front porch exposing your skin to bright sunlight (and to your nosey neighbors) on a daily basis, you will probably need to be taking an oral supplement to maintain your vitamin D level in the ideal range. The average American gets a paltry 150 IU daily of vitamin D from foods in their diet and the typical multivitamin provides only about 400 IUs of vitamin D_3.

Important research hot off the press: a study published in July 5, 2012, issue of *The New England Journal of Medicine* found that vitamin D_3, when taken in higher doses—between 800 and 2,000 IUs per day—substantially reduces the likelihood of broken bones in both men and women. This was a meta-analysis of 11 individual randomized controlled trials all of which focused on the effect of vitamin D_3 supplementation in those over age 65. Among the 31,000 seniors who were taking between 800 to 2,000 IU of vitamin D_3, they found a 30 percent decrease in the risk of hip fractures with a significant decrease in risk of fractures of other bones as well. However, the researchers found no significant reduction in fracture risk for doses of vitamin D less than 800 IUs daily.

Based on this study and a growing body of research we recommend that you consume about 2,000 IU of vitamin D_3 per day. Many individuals need more than this to keep their blood levels of vitamin D in the ideal range of 30 to 60 ng/ml. Vitamin D is not only critical for bone strength—as this important new research shows, but it may also reduce risks for many of the most common serious diseases including diabetes, high blood pressure, cancer, heart disease, and autoimmune disorders. Alarmingly, vitamin D deficiency is an epidemic in America, with up to 2 out of 3 of us having suboptimal levels of this critically important compound. Some experts have estimated that up to a third of cancer cases might be avoided if we all consumed adequate amounts of vitamin D on a daily basis.

You do not need to worry that 2,000 IU will be an excessive dose. When you go outside in a bathing suit and bask in the summer sunlight, your skin will make about 10,000 IU to 20,000 IU of vitamin D per hour with no chance of creating vitamin D toxicity. Additionally, studies indicate that vitamin D supplements at doses of up to 5,000 IU daily seem to be safe—although we don't recommend taking these high doses unless your vitamin D blood levels are being monitored. One more point: to ensure maximal absorption, try to consume your vitamin D with a meal that contains some healthy fat like olive oil, fish oil, nuts, or avocados.

Joan, like many women, was plagued with recurrent urinary tract infections (UTIs) for years. It got to the point that she was on antibiotics almost every month for a UTI. It was making her miserable and dejected; and it worried us both, what with the frequent courses of antibiotics, which kill off the pathogens (disease-causing microbes) but also eliminate the friendly bacteria that are so essential for healthy gastrointestinal function and an optimal immune system. Chronic antibiotic use predisposes to all sorts of problems, such as yeast infections, GI upset, and the emergence of 'super-bugs' in your system that have developed resistance to most or all antibiotics. And since Joan had her spleen removed when she had cancer during her first pregnancy, any infection can be a potentially life-threatening problem for her. She saw several physicians about this, and tried various tactics: cranberry juice, prophylactic antibiotics, increasing intake of fluids, but nothing seemed to work.

Then, as we became aware of the many important benefits of normalizing vitamin D levels, including strengthened immunity, she started 2,000 IU of vitamin D_3 (a modest dose by current standards, but at that time, 10 times the Recommended Daily Intake of 200 IU). Joan noticed that the UTIs seemed to be occurring less frequently, but were still a problem, so she increased her daily dose to 4,000 IU of vitamin D_3. The UTIs were now markedly decreased but still occurred occasionally. Finally, she increased her daily dose of vitamin D_3 to 6,000 IU, and the UTIs miraculously disappeared entirely! And when we measured her vitamin D blood levels on the 6,000 IU per day (10 times the recently updated Recommended Daily Intake of 600 IU according to the Institute of Medicine) we found them to be about 60 ng/ml, which is upper range of what is considered ideal.

We have shared this recommendation for higher dose vitamin D_3 with many other women who have been tormented by recurring UTIs, and they have generally noted similar improvements in their resistance to infections. The dramatic protection against UTIs is just one readily apparent manifestation of vitamin D induced bolstering of the power of the immune system. Studies show that vitamin D is important for not only improving the vigilance of the immune system—its ability to recognize foreign invaders whether they be cancer cells or dangerous microbes—but also its ability to kill these potentially lethal threats. Indeed, research shows that keeping your vitamin D levels well in the normal levels may reduce risks for many of the most common and lethal malignancies, including melanoma, and cancers of the colon, breast, and prostate.

My grandfather, Dr. Emmet O'Keefe, as you may recall, contracted tuberculosis from one of his patients shortly after he finished his training. At one point he was so close to death due to "the consumption" (the common name for TB in centuries past) that my grandmother was told to go home and pick out the suit in which she wanted him to be buried the next day. But he survived that crisis, and shortly thereafter, in 1932, he was admitted to a TB sanatorium. These were hospitals where patients with TB were exposed to fresh air each day, typically by rolling their beds out onto an open air veranda. Although the physicians thought it was something about the fresh air that helped to cure their patients' TB, they were doing the right thing for the wrong reason. The curative factor in the outdoor therapy was the sunshine's UV light radiating down on the skin of the TB victim, immediately raising the vitamin D levels. A normal vitamin D level endows a person with a much stronger immune system, thus giving him a fighting chance of eradicating the notoriously resistant and virulent tuberculosis infections, even without antibiotics (which of course were not available only a few generations ago). When he contracted TB, my grandfather was certain to be profoundly vitamin D deficient, what with working indoors and living near the Canadian border in North Dakota. Had he not been moved to the sanatorium in the sunny climate, where he bathed in the immune-bolstering solar radiation each day for months, he would have almost certainly succumbed to the consumption.

We wrote a paper with Drs. Michael Horlicks, Chip Lavie, and David Bell, that was published in the *Journal of the American College of Cardiology*, proposing that vitamin D deficiency is a common and important cardiovascular risk factor. Our skin manufactures this vitamin D in response to the UV-B light rays present in sunlight. In the past, humans naturally kept their vitamin D levels in the healthy range just by being outside in the sunshine, and consuming a diet high in ocean fish. But these days even in the non-winter months, with our indoor lifestyles and occupations, and sun-protected clothing and sunscreens when we are outside, many of us are vitamin D deficient. If you live north of a line between Atlanta to Phoenix to Los Angeles, you will have a hard time maintaining normal vitamin D levels in the months from September through April, even if you spend quite a lot of time outside.

This vitamin is really more of a hormone due to its wide-ranging effects throughout the body. We have known for a long time that vitamin D is important for building and maintaining strong bones and muscles. However, vitamin D receptors are not just in present in our musculoskeletal system, but also are in the heart and blood vessels, the kidneys, pancreas, white blood cells, and brain. Low vitamin D levels predispose to high blood pressure, diabetes, inflammation, and adverse cardiovascular events such as heart attack and stroke. Additionally, vitamin D deficiency has been strongly linked to many types of cancers, and infections, in addition to inflammatory and/or auto-immune diseases such as multiple sclerosis and Alzheimer's disease.

Make sure you have your vitamin D level tested. If it is low, work with your doctor to get it back into the normal range. The current recommendations for suggested daily vitamin D_3 intake of about 600 to 800 IU per day are far too low. The average American consumes about 200 IU per day of vitamin D, and yet a consensus statement of experts recently recommended that most Americans need at least 10 times that much, or 2,000 IU of vitamin D_3 daily. Most of us are deficient in this crucially important nutrient. Importantly, getting outside on a daily basis for about 15 to 20 minutes of sensible sunlight is a splendid strategy to naturally boost your vitamin D levels.

Rose's Green Tea

My great-grandmother, Rose Cartier, grew up in Montreal, Canada. We called her Ma Mère (French for "my mother"), and I recall her as a delightful lady with a loving disposition, a stout constitution, and a mind that remained sharp and active throughout her long life. She took pleasure in chatting with her family and friends; and spoke French when discussing issues with my grandmother and my mother that she didn't want to share with us kids. At age 94, after a full and contented life, Rose went to bed one evening, fell asleep peacefully, and just never woke up. Even as a child, I remember thinking, what a great way to live... and die.

The only medication she took regularly was aspirin, for her rheumatism. Rose loved good food, and enjoyed a glass of red wine before her evening meal. Yet, it was her tea—green tea specifically—that was her defining habit. Rose would always have loose leaf green tea steeping in a ceramic white teapot that sat on the kitchen table. I recall her playfully reading the tea leaves at the bottom of our cups to "tell the future." If you want your future health to be bright and rosy, I would suggest that you take a cue from my great-grandmother, and make tea (green tea whenever possible) one of your beverages of choice. The accumulating scientific evidence indicates Rose's daily habit of drinking green tea probably played a big role in why she was so healthy, happy, and clever for almost a century.

People who make a habit of drinking 4 or more cups of green tea daily are 44 percent less likely to suffer from depression. Theanine may be the reason; this is a unique amino acid present in green tea that induces a mental state of relaxed awareness, increasing alertness while at the same time reducing anxiety. Heavily caffeinated beverages like Red Bull, Monster, Rockstar, and 5-Hour Energy, especially in excess, will make you jittery and anxious, and are implicated as a cause heart attack, stroke, and death (even in teenagers). On the other hand, agents that reduce anxiety, like alcohol or Xanax, tend to reduce your energy level, make you feel fatigued, and, in massive overdoses, can kill you. But if you are looking for a natural and safe boost to your mental alertness and energy that will also leave you feeling relaxed and focused, green tea is your drink.

Many recent studies have focused on the health effects of drinking coffee and tea, and the results are generally encouraging. The research shows that a routine of 2 to 4 cups of coffee per day is linked with lower risks of heart disease, diabetes, depression, and Parkinson's disease, and a slightly reduced risk of death from all causes. Tea consumption has also been linked to powerful health benefits. For instance, drinking 3 to 6 cups of tea daily is associated with a 45 percent lower risk of death from heart disease. Long-term generous consumption of tea has also been shown to lower blood pressure and improve cholesterol levels. Studies suggest that green tea might play a role in preventing Alzheimer's disease, macular degeneration (the most common cause of blindness in adults), and several cancers including cancers of the mouth, lung, prostate, and leukemia. Tea can aid digestion, strengthen bones, and improve the health of gums and teeth. Frequent tea consumption is linked to better longevity. In a study of 40,000 Japanese followed for 11 years, results showed that those who drank green tea on a daily basis were less likely to die from all causes, and seemed to be especially protected from cardiovascular death.

A study focusing on Chinese people offered fascinating insight into how tea might improve longevity. Men who consumed 3 or more cups of tea daily were genetically younger than those who consumed less tea. In this study, the tea drinkers had significantly longer telomeres. Avid tea drinkers' telomeres showed substantially less wear and tear, translating into a genetic age about 5 years younger than the non-tea drinkers.

Drinking a lot of tea can be helpful if you are trying to lose weight. Besides being a tasty and healthy calorie-free drink, tea also cranks up your metabolism which burns off belly fat. Studies show that drinking at least 3 or 4 cups of tea, especially green tea, will help to flatten your tummy and trim your waistline—which is not only great for your figure, but also for your health.

The health benefits of tea may be due to the high levels of antioxidants and other plant chemicals in the beverage. Studies show that you tend to absorb more of these beneficial antioxidants from your tea if you add a slice or squeeze of lemon. Tea, whether iced or hot, green or black, is naturally calorie free. Try to learn to enjoy your tea unsweetened; both sugar and artificial sweeteners make it a less healthy beverage. Your abdominal fat will really melt away if you substitute green tea for soda and other sweet drinks.

Bottom line: try to include tea in your daily routine. Green tea and white tea are probably best for health benefits; and if caffeine bothers you, drink the decaf versions. Or, if you just can't or won't drink green tea regularly, consider taking a daily supplement, in the form a capsule of tea antioxidants. Getting your tea antioxidants in the form of a daily capsule has been shown to significantly lower cholesterol and blood pressure, and help to trim excess belly fat.

I have been impressed that my patients, family, and friends seem to feel better and be healthier when they add either green tea or a tea supplement to their daily routine. Joan has a hard time drinking as much tea as she needs, so she takes 2 capsules of green tea supplement, which she swears helps her to keep her girlish figure and small waistline. If we are out of her tea supplement, Joan sends me to the store to get some immediately. It is her secret weapon for fighting belly fat and staying young. As for me, I'm following Ma Mère's example and drinking at least 4 cups of green tea daily; and I enjoy it as much as she did, though I brew mine from tea bags, so I'm unable see the future from the tea leaves like she could.

CHAPTER 15

Achieve Ideal Cholesterol Levels without Drugs

Natural, Over-the-Counter Cholesterol Lowering Strategies

Several natural, over-the-counter therapies are available for lowering your bad cholesterol. Consider using these options listed below, if you can't or don't need to take a prescription statin but still would like to help keep your cholesterol levels in the ideal ranges. It is always a good idea to discuss these issues with your doctor to be sure we are doing what's best for you in the long run.

Soluble Fiber

Soluble fiber dissolves in water into a gel that helps to prevent cholesterol absorption from the food you eat. Soluble fiber is present in many plant foods including broccoli, apples, oatmeal, carrots, plums, prunes, pears, citrus fruits (oranges, grapefruit, and lemons, etc.), beans, and nuts. Psyllium, the plant that is used in most fiber supplements including Metamucil, Fiber One, and Citrucel, is also high in soluble fiber. Adding soluble fiber to your diet is an underrated way to lower the bad cholesterol. For her clients who are trying to lower their cholesterol, Joan routinely recommends 1 heaping tablespoon of Metamucil stirred into at least 16 ounces of water once daily. By the way, you will want to drink this immediately after mixing, before it has time to turn to a gel-like consistency.

If you can drink your Metamucil once daily it will lower your LDL about 6 percent. If you can do it 3 times per day (not likely to happen for most people) it will lower LDL by 10 to 15 percent. Metamucil is also helpful if you are trying to lose excess weight, in which case you should consume the 1 heaping tablespoon mixed into 16 ounces of cold water and downed just before your evening meal. One heaping tablespoon of Metamucil contains 6 grams of fiber. If you are working on getting down to ideal weight, it is best to use the artificially sweetened or unsweetened varieties of Metamucil. Joan recommends Metamucil to virtually all of her clients, whether it's for lowering cholesterol naturally or helping with weight loss, however, soluble fiber is also is also great for the health of your gastro-intestinal tract. It is for this reason that one of her client refers to her as the Colon Queen. A high intake of soluble fiber will clear up constipation and help to prevent problems such as irritable bowel. Just be sure to take the Metamucil with plenty of water or it can cause constipation; and if you get diarrhea, lower the dose or stop it altogether.

Plant Sterols

Plant Sterols, also called phytosterols, are natural products that come from plants such as nuts, beans, and vegetable oils. Plant sterols lower blood cholesterol by reducing the amount of cholesterol you absorb from your food. Plant sterols have been used for almost 2 decades now and are the most extensively tested over-the-counter therapy for lowering cholesterol. Four capsules per day of CardioSterol, either all at once or 2 caps twice daily will lower your bad cholesterol about 10 to 12 percent. Plant sterols have virtually no side effects, and although you can get them in the form of margarines, you will have to consume about 2 tablespoons of the spread and a lot of calories to get the full cholesterol lowering dose of 1.3 to 2 grams of phytosterols. That is why we recommend you get the plant sterols from a diet high in plants and CardioSterol capsules.

Vitamin D

We discussed this earlier, but let's talk about its benefits for people on cholesterol-lowering medications. The first symptom of vitamin D deficiency is aches and pains in the muscles, joints, and bones. Restoring vitamin D levels to normal will not only allow many people to take a statin who otherwise could not, it may also cool off inflammation, lower blood pressure, and reduce the risk of diabetes. Ask your doctor to check your vitamin D level.

Tea Supplements

I hope I have made it clear from the earlier stories, that tea can provide real health benefits, including lowering cholesterol. The antioxidant compounds that occur naturally in tea have been shown to be modestly effective in lowering LDL cholesterol.

Fish Oil

Fish oil is one of the most crucial supplements to consume, as I've addressed earlier. It's important enough to remind you here that the omega-3 fats found in fish oil are very effective for lowering bad blood lipids including triglycerides and non-HDL cholesterol, as well as raising the good cholesterol, HDL. To get these benefits, you will need to take a moderate to high dose of omega-3.

Red Yeast Rice

My brother Kevin is typical of many people. When he takes a statin to lower his high cholesterol, his muscles ache and he feels generally unwell. Over the past 2 decades, he has tried taking various statins on at least a dozen different occasions. Each time he tries one, the medication does a marvelous job of getting his cholesterol down to a much healthier level, but after a few weeks he begins to feel soreness in his muscles and joints.

I suggest to him that maybe it's all in his head, and he tells me, "No James, it's actually all in my neck—aching pain and stiffness, every time you insist I take one of those prescription statins." But Kevin's cholesterol level, when he's off a statin, runs about 240, despite following a healthy diet and lifestyle. And to make matters worse, a few years ago we discovered a moderate amount of plaque in his coronary arteries on a CardioScan screening. So it really is critically important that we get his cholesterol down, way down, to less than 160 ideally.

Thankfully, we now have safe and natural over-the-counter (OTC) options for people like Kevin who can't or won't take a statin, and for others with high cholesterol, but who are at lower risk and thus may not need the potency of a prescription drug. The most effective OTC option for lowering cholesterol is Red Yeast Rice, a product of a fungus (monascus purpureus) grown on rice. The first documentation of the use of Red Yeast Rice was in China during the Tang Dynasty 1,200 year ago, where it was recommended for a variety of ailments such as poor blood circulation and indigestion. Red Yeast Rice contains natural compounds called monacolins, which are quite effective at inhibiting cholesterol production by the liver. In the late 1970s, scientists isolated monacolin-K, later renamed lovastatin, from a fungus. This was concentrated and purified and in 1987 lovastatin was approved and marketed by Merck as the first statin, which subsequently has grown into the largest selling class of prescription drugs in the history. Because Red Yeast Rice contains a much lower concentration of monacolins compared to prescription statins, they tend to be much easier to tolerate with fewer side effects.

Studies from Dr. David Becker and others show that Red Yeast Rice can lower the bad (LDL) cholesterol about 20 percent by itself, or up to 40 percent (or as good as simvastatin) when it is combined with high-dose omega-3. Even more encouraging are studies from China showing that Red Yeast Rice, like statins, may reduce heart attacks and cardiac deaths. The largest of these studies, the China Coronary Secondary Prevention Study, randomized 5,000 people who had suffered a heart attack to Red Yeast Rice or a placebo (inactive look-alike) pill. After 4½ years the people on the Red Yeast Rice suffered 45 percent fewer heart attacks and 33 percent fewer deaths compared to the group on the placebo. The Red Yeast Rice therapy was safe and well tolerated in this large study.

However, there is a dark side to Red Yeast Rice. Nearly all of it is produced in China, frequently in facilities that would not meet FDA standards for safety or purity. Sometimes Red Yeast Rice of Chinese origin can contain citrinin, a dangerous chemical that is toxic to kidneys. And other times it can be laced with a pharmaceutical-strength statin, and thus the unsuspecting consumer might actually be taking a highly potent statin despite buying OTC Red Yeast Rice.

The solution is to use a Red Yeast Rice product that is safe, effective and produced under highly regulated conditions. The standard dose of Red Yeast Rice is 2 to 4 600 mg capsules per day (1,200 to 2,400 mg total per day). You can expect that this will lower your bad LDL cholesterol by 15 to 20 percent. I frequently see patients in whom Red Yeast Rice dropped their bad cholesterol from 130 down to 100 or less.

If you want to get the benefits of cholesterol lowering, you have to stick with the therapy for the long-term, years to even decades. In order to do that, whatever therapy you take can't make you feel miserable. If you are someone who needs a lower cholesterol, but can't tolerate the statins, or someone without heart disease who doesn't want to resort to prescription medicines, consider Red Yeast Rice in combination with a high quality omega-3 supplement, and make it a priority to eat right and exercise each day. This is a strategy for impressive cholesterol numbers and a healthy heart today and for decades to come.

Five Strategies to Boost Your HDL

Good cholesterol (HDL) is helpful in preventing plaque buildup and heart attacks. We have great medications (principally the statin drugs) for lowering the LDL cholesterol. However, the pharmacologic options for raising HDL levels are much more limited.

Certainly, your HDL is strongly influenced by your genes, yet lifestyle and diet are also very important in determining your HDL level. The bottom line is that although your HDL level is a crucial number in predicting your long-term health and longevity, at least for the next several years, boosting this level into a healthy range is mostly up to you. Here's what works.

1. <u>Curb the carbs</u>. Eliminate sugar and other processed carbohydrates like white bread, rolls, white flour, white rice, cookies, and other sweets. These high-glycemic index foods spike triglycerides and blood sugar and drag your HDL down.

2. <u>Change your oil</u>. The omega-3 fats in fish oil can raise HDL about 8 percent. Other healthy oils that foster higher HDL levels can be found in natural foods like avocados, ground flaxseed, extra virgin olive oil, green leafy vegetables, and nuts (especially tree nuts like walnuts, pecans, almonds, and Brazil nuts). On the other hand, trans fats, like those in French fries and commercial baked goods, will lower the protective HDL levels.

3. <u>Achieve and maintain a healthy weight</u>. Excess body fat, especially around the waist, will depress your HDL, and increase your risks for diabetes, heart attack and stroke. For every 6 pounds of excess weight you can shed, your HDL will rise 1 mg/dl.

4. <u>Clean up your act</u>. Smoking tobacco will lower your HDL by about 10 percent; whereas kicking this lethal habit will quickly

bounce your HDL back up to baseline. Drinking 1 alcoholic drink per day will raise your HDL by about 10 percent. More alcohol will raise your HDL even more, but will increase your risk for other problems like cancer, stroke, and accidents.

5. <u>Move your body</u>. Exercise, especially aerobic exercise like walking, running, swimming, and cycling, will raise the HDL level in a dose-dependent fashion—the more exercise you do, and the more intense the effort, the higher your HDL will rise. Ideally, we like to see people exercising aerobically 30 to 50 minutes daily, and doing strength training at least 20 to 30 minutes at least twice weekly.

CHAPTER 16

Safely Harnessing the Power of Modern Pharmaceuticals

The Pharmaceutical Industry Can Be Your Ally

I am bothered by occasional, irregular, or 'skipped' heartbeats at random times during the day. For quite a while I tried to ignore it, hoping it would disappear, but it didn't and the palpitations, as we call them, started to really distract and worry me. So I saw a cardiologist (I bump into one of those types about every 10 minutes during a typical workday). My good friend put me through the standard cardiology routine—EKG, echo stress imaging study, and blood work. The tests all turned out fine, but I was still tormented by irregular heartbeats.

Those of you who know me understand that I really prefer to treat medical problems as naturally as possible. For years, I have been diligent about following a regimen of daily exercise and a very healthy diet (thanks in large part to Joan). I also take vitamin D_3, omega-3, and a statin. However, my cardiologist-friend suggested I try a beta blocker on an as-needed basis for the palpitations. I was a bit skeptical because these medicines are notorious for causing side effects like fatigue; but I was distressed about the palpitations so I gave it a try. Within 24 hours of starting a low dose of carvedilol, the palpitations virtually vanished. I was relieved and grateful to have a safe and effective pharmacologic solution to the problem that, while not life-threatening, was still very upsetting. I still use low dose carvedilol when I feel my palpitations flaring up.

This episode gave me a new, very personal appreciation for the power of modern pharmacology. Life expectancy has almost doubled over the past century in America. Scientists who have studied this phenomenon attribute most of these gains in longevity to the vast and potent armamentarium of pharmacologic agents we have at our disposal that can, for example, eradicate infections, reverse heart disease, and treat and usually cure most cancers.

Yet, the prescription drug industry today has a serious image problem. Indeed, a recent public opinion poll about the trustworthiness of various American business sectors placed the pharmaceutical industry near the bottom of the list; just 1 step above the tobacco and oil industries. Some of this concern is warranted, but too often worried patients abruptly stop their drugs without consulting with their health care providers, which sometimes leaves them with dangerously uncontrolled medical problems such as diabetes, high blood pressure, or high cholesterol. Most of drugs we commonly use in cardiology have been so extensively tested that we have a high level of confidence in their safety and effectiveness. If you have concerns about your medications, please discuss them with your health care providers. We can either reassure you about their safety or find an alternative treatment for you.

We like to emphasize the importance of taking advantage of the best of both worlds. It is essential that you do your best to take care of yourself by following our advice about lifestyle and diet. But often that is not enough to keep you completely healthy. When you decide to go it alone and shun prescription drugs, you are depriving yourself of one of the powerful advantages of living in the 21st century.

With respect to health issues, most people cruise along pretty smoothly down the road of life in their youth, but by middle age the ride can start to get bumpy. Ignore major issues and by the time you get into the decades of your 50s or 60s (and sometimes even sooner) the wheels may just come off and your life will grind to a halt. By using the natural therapies first and adding the high-tech modern therapies when needed, we can almost always get you back up to speed and ready to live life with gusto again.

The future will hold even more spectacular pharmacologic fixes. Be smart about working with your health care providers to take advantage of the therapies you may need to ensure your ride along your journey through life is as smooth and trouble-free as possible. I was chatting with a hospitalized patient whose kidneys had recently failed, "Well, Wayne, what did you think of your first dialysis session?" He shrugged, rolled his eyes, and said cynically, "I could live without it." I replied, "No, Wayne, actually, you could not live without it."

How to Save Your Life for 11 Cents a Day!

One of my patients told me, "My wife got the medications mixed up around our household earlier this week. So the dog has been dragging around with low blood pressure; and you can be assured that I will be heartworm-free for at least the next 30 days." In truth most Americans, by the time they reach middle age, need 1 or more prescription meds to keep their crucial health care numbers in the ideal ranges.

Julia is thrilled that her insurance company will send her a 90-day supply of generic Norvasc (amlodipine) for just $40. What she doesn't know is that she could take that same prescription down to her local discount pharmacy and pick up a 90-day supply for just $10. In fact, for many of the medicines we most commonly prescribe you are better off pretending that you don't have prescription coverage from your insurance company at all, and instead just purchase a 30 or 90-day supply and paying for it out-of-pocket, assuming you do your homework and find a pharmacy that sells generics at deeply discounted prices.

There is a silver lining behind the storm clouds that are threatening to make modern medical care unaffordable; powerful market forces are driving the prices of many first-rate medications to remarkably inexpensive levels. Each year more and more of the very best drugs for improving cardiovascular health, and extending your longevity, are becoming available as inexpensive generics, often for as little as $4 a month or $10 for a 90-day supply. Generic drugs now account for about 80 percent of all prescriptions written by U.S. physicians.

The skyrocketing popularity of generic drugs is due to the fact that they provide the same benefits as the original brand-name medicines at a fraction of the price. This is causing serious financial pain for the big pharmaceutical corporations as sales of their billion dollar blockbuster drugs vanish almost overnight when cheap generic copycats become available. Nonetheless, between 1996 and 2006, the percent of income spent on prescription drugs doubled to about 18 percent for the average American.

When it comes to prescription drugs, you don't necessarily get what you pay for. Even inexpensive generics have to pass muster with the FDA and prove that they provide as much active medication as the name-brand drug. Typically a drug will have 10 to 15 years of exclusive sales before its patent expires. When a brand-name drug loses its patent protection, generic drug companies are free to manufacture and market a duplicate of the drug. By FDA standards a generic drug must be bioequivalent, meaning that after it is swallowed, it will reliably produce blood levels similar to those produced by the brand-name drug. Sure, the generic drug may contain some different inactive ingredients, and hence the pill may be of a different size, color, shape, or taste compared to the brand-name version—but by law its active ingredients must be the same. About 4 out of 5 prescriptions I write are specified as 'substitution permitted,' meaning a generic substitution is allowable. Just pay attention to the pharmaceutical company that makes the drug you are using, and try to be consistent about sticking with that same brand, assuming it's seeming to work well for you.

Generic Life-Saving Medications—Wonder Drugs at Wonderful Prices

If you are on expensive name brand drugs, ask your doctor and/or pharmacist if 1 of these might be an option for you:

- Chlorthalidone (Hygroton), or Indapamide (Lozol). Two highly effective diuretics (pills for eliminating excess fluid from your system), typically used for high blood pressure.

- Atorvastatin (Lipitor) or Simvastatin (Zocor). Cholesterol-lowering statin drugs proven to prevent heart attacks and save lives.

- Clopidogrel (Plavix). Anti-platelet drugs to prevent blood clots, heart attacks, and strokes, especially for a person with 1 or more stents in their arteries.

- Metformin (Glucophage). A safe and effective medication for diabetes.

- Perindopril (Aceon) or Lisinopril (Prinivil). This class of meds, called the ACE Inhibitors, is proven and safe blood pressure lowering therapy. Lisinopril is the most commonly prescribed blood pressure pill.

- Carvedilol (Coreg). A phenomenally effective drug for treating heart disease, heart failure, high blood pressure, and heart rhythm problems. Truly a life-saving therapy for many individuals.

- Amlodipine (Norvasc). A highly effective blood pressure drug, especially good for preventing stokes.

Public Enemy #1: Addictive, Mind-Altering Prescription Drugs

Although America's "war on drugs" is aimed at the illegal street drugs like cocaine, marijuana, and methamphetamine, legal prescription drugs today kill many more people. The latest data from U.S. Centers for Disease Control and Prevention (CDC) showed that for the first time in history, Americans are now more likely to die from prescription drugs than motor vehicle accidents. The availability of inexpensive generics is a mixed blessing. For a few dollars a month we can purchase life-saving medicines like atorvastatin, amlodipine, carvedilol, and indapamide; but we also have ready access to many other highly addictive, mind-altering, potentially dangerous drugs like oxycodone, hydrocodone, alprazolam, Ambien, and Ativan.

In 2009, 36,300 people died in traffic accidents compared with 37,500 people who died from prescription drugs, predominantly due to overdoses of medications for pain and anxiety such as OxyContin, Vicodin, Xanax, and Soma. Additionally, in 2009, adverse reactions to drugs accounted for approximately 4.6 million visits to hospital emergency departments.

The death rate is highest among individuals in their 40s, but everyone from teenagers to the elderly are falling victim to these dangerous and highly addictive drugs. Indeed, studies show that prescription drugs are now the preferred "high" for many individuals, especially teenagers, because drugs are often readily available in the medicine cabinets of most homes these days.

Generally, many people start off using these pain relievers, anti-anxiety drugs, or sleep aids for legitimate problems like headaches, depression, or back pain, but can become addicted. These prescription medicines are particularly lethal when used in combination with alcoholic beverages.

During unusually difficult times, temporary use of these medicines can reduce suffering. But be careful: these drugs are highly addictive. When you get a prescription for relief of pain, anxiety, or insomnia, use as few pills as possible and dispose of any leftovers. Stress, anxiety, and pain are unavoidable in life. Rather than routinely resorting to mind-altering prescription drugs for stress reduction, sleeplessness, and pain relief, it is important to develop healthy coping strategies such as outdoor walking or other forms of exercise that you find fun and relaxing, playing with friends and family, meditation, social support groups, yoga, getting enough sleep, religious services, psychological counseling, and confiding in your loved ones. It is essential that you have several effective options for diffusing stress by constructive, healthy, and non-pharmaceutical means.

Prayer comforts many people, but it can also lower one's blood pressure. By simply meditating quietly, especially if you take slow, deep breaths, and focus on prolonging the exhalation phase (breathing out) you can slow your pulse and lower your blood pressure. Similar to prayer, relaxation breathing can reduce stress and is easy to do: breathe in for the count of 4, hold your breath for the count of 7, and breathe out slowly for the count of 8. Even doing just 4 to 8 cycles of this relaxation breathing will lower your blood pressure and reduce your sense of anxiety.

PART II

CHAPTER 17

Good Things First: The Recipe for Raising Healthy and Happy Kids

The Hazards of Growing up in 21st Century America

To us, children are the joy and the light of the world. Their eyes sparkle with energy and curiosity, and the future belongs to them. By nature, we are hard-wired to worry about the safety and well-being of our children and grandchildren. We put so much time, effort, and love into raising these kids; in them we invest our hopes and dreams. So we buckle them in, smear on the sunscreen, strap on their helmets, and supervise their every move like watchful mother hens. Yet many parents unwittingly poison their children on a daily basis by giving them drive-thru junk food and unlimited access to inactive pastimes like TV, computer games, and spectator sports.

Indeed, the modern world is a very dangerous place in which to grow up, but not for the reasons about which most parents fret. To be sure, abductions, accidents, violent deaths, serious infections, and child abuse are tragic events that still scar or end too many young lives. Yet the likelihood that a newborn baby will grow safely into maturity is far better today than it has ever been in the history of humankind. Stephen Pinker in his tour de force *The Better Angels of Our Nature: Why Violence Has Declined* calculated that if a parent was trying to get his kid abducted, statistically speaking, the child would have to be left unattended on a street corner for about 750,000 years. Clearly, we have more pressing concerns about our children than cloistering them away indoors in front of a screen lest they be kidnapped by a stranger.

The Biggest Threats to Our Children

The more insidious dangers that stalk our children are disguised as harmless pleasures: way too little physical play and fresh air, and way too much TV and junk food. Diabetes, depression, and obesity increasingly threaten to ruin the health and longevity of the new generation. Obesity among children has risen 5-fold in just 25 years, and experts predict that ⅓ to ½ of all American children born in the new millennium will develop diabetes in their lifetime.

These calamities result from a diet and lifestyle that are increasingly at odds with our genetic identity. Kids were meant to be very physically active. The single best predictor of mood in a long-term studies of teenagers is their level of daily physical exercise—inactive kids tend to be depressed, whereas active youngsters tend to be happy. The most important step you can take to ensure the long-term vitality, both emotional and physical, of the children in your life, is by teaching them by example how to eat right and find their fun mostly through physical play.

Outdoor exercise was, by necessity, how all humans stayed fit for countless millennia. However, in recent decades most people have migrated indoors permanently, transitioning abruptly into an unnatural mole-like existence. Yet the natural world remains our native milieu and it has the power to energize and inspire our lives. The vogue terms for outdoor activities are *ecotherapy* or *green exercise*, and we are enthusiastic advocates of this fitness strategy for kids.

An English team of researchers recently reported that a 30-minute walk in a park boosted self-esteem and lifted depression, whereas a half-hour stroll in a mall actually *increased* tension. We can personally attest to the fact that when we want to relax, an indoor mall would be about the last place we would think of going. On the other hand, we find that walking outdoors with the kids through the Plaza in Kansas City, for example, to be invigorating and fun. Even more enjoyable is an outing to Loose Park with the kids and dogs to spend an hour walking, running, scooting, skating, climbing trees, or playing Frisbee.

If you could see what was happening in your kid's or grand-kid's bloodstream and arteries right after they gulp down a Happy Meal, it would make you cringe. A fast food meal of a cheeseburger, fries, and a Coke will cause dangerous rises in the blood levels of glucose and fats that immediately trigger inflammation, stress hormone release, a rise in blood pressure, and constriction of the blood vessels—even in apparently healthy young people. In fact, the stress to the arteries induced by such a meal is the same as smoking 2 cigarettes. So when you take your kids out for a burger, fries, and a shake, you might as well be taking them out behind the garage to teach them how to inhale cigarettes. Do everything you can to see that the kids in your life eat more natural, unprocessed whole foods like vegetables, fruits, nuts, and berries and fresh wholesome protein sources, and less of the ubiquitous tasty, but toxic junk food.

Nature's Candy

We have always thought of berries as nature's candy, and they are 1 of our kids' favorite foods. By nature, children have a powerful 'sweet-tooth.' Natural sweetness is a marker of a high-calorie treat that can fuel the energetic pursuits of youth. Berries occupy 6 of the top 10 spots on the list of the best antioxidant foods, including tangy and tasty options such as wild blueberries, regular (cultivated) blueberries, strawberries, blackberries, and raspberries.

The Recipe for Raising an Exceptional Child

1. No eating in front of a screen, no exceptions, no negotiations. Mindless eating while watching TV or playing on a computer nearly always involves junk food, and too much of it.

2. When introducing nutritious foods that your child is not accustomed to eating, give him or her 1 bite on the dinner plate. Expecting your kid to eat a whole serving of broccoli right from the get-go you is just inviting strife to the dinner table. Family meal time should be for bonding, not fighting, so ask them to eat 1 bite, with 1 stipulation, "No treats after dinner if you don't finish your meal." If they chose to not eat it, but want a treat afterwards, remind them of the 'Good Things First' motto and them tell them in a kind yet firm tone, "You are done eating for the evening." It may take 10 tries before you get them to eat that first bite, but with time 1 bite turns into 2, then 3, then 4. Don't give up; if you don't pick the battle of developing your child's taste for healthy food it is not going to happen. Using this strategy, Joan has turned each of our 4 children into lovers of vegetables, fish, seafood, and fruits. When the kids complain too much about the nutritious food around our house we jokingly tell them "the beatings will continue until the morale improves." Keep in mind that you only have until they get their driver's license to instill these eating habits, at which point they are mobile and on their own in a world where junk food is tempting them everywhere they go.

3. They are watching you—so you need the walk the walk. Evan's first word was 'bean'; when Evan was a baby Joan's favorite food was a marinated bean salad. She would throw a few beans onto his high-chair tray and he would gobble them down. Don't expect them to eat foods you refuse to eat, or tell them to avoid fast food and sweet beverages while you indulge in these unhealthy choices yourself. Your kids are not going to eat unsweetened Greek yogurt for breakfast while you are shoveling Coco Puffs into your mouth.

4. Avoid sweet drinks for your kids… no juices, no sodas, no sports drinks, no milk shakes, no sweetened coffees or teas, no energy drinks. Skim or 1 percent milk is important for bone-building in children and adolescents. Chocolate low-fat milk is the perfect sports recovery drink; a better option than the slickly marketed beverages like Gatorade and Powerade.

5. Feed your children a healthy breakfast each morning that is rich in fiber and contains a serving of protein. This type of meal is digested slowly, ensuring steady and normal blood sugar levels throughout the morning which will allow them to focus, learn, and test well right up until noon. A high-carb breakfast of pancakes, waffles, toast, sweet cereal, doughnuts, orange juice, and the like will spike your child's blood sugar 30 to 60 minutes later, followed by an abrupt crash that makes it almost impossible to concentrate. Also, hypoglycemia stimulates hunger and adrenalin which render many children and adolescents hyperactive, distractible, and virtually un-teachable.

6. Joan says "Put them to bed! It's good for them, it's good for you. Don't take no for an answer—they need their sleep." Sleep helps kids to grow, learn, and test optimally. Sleep needs to be prioritized above TV, gaming, texting, social engagements, and even above sports and homework. Inadequate sleep in kids has been linked to obesity, lower test scores, shorter stature and emotional explosions. The following is a general guide to sleep needs among kids of various ages according to WebMD.

    3 to 6 Years Old: 10 to 12 hours per night

    7 to 12 Years Old: 10 to 11 hours per night

    12 to 18 Years Old: 8 to 9 hours per night

7. Strike when the iron is hot. When Joan picks the kids up at school they tend to be hungry and cranky, so she always has a bowl of strawberries or some other fruit waiting for them in the

back seat. By the time they get home they are happier, less famished, and more reasonable about what they want to eat next.

8. When your young daughter complains "I'm hungry," only give her choices with which you will be happy. So you say "How about an apple, or some nuts, or some grapes?" When she says "I want chips," you reply, "Good things first. Have some fruit or nuts and then we will talk."

9. Make your home a safe place for eating. Do not bring home options that you don't want your child to have. Any treat should have some redeeming value—like dark chocolate covered almonds, nutritious popcorn (not microwave) or dried mango slices.

10. Children and adolescents need at least 1 hour of vigorous physical activity on most days, according to the U.S. Centers for Disease Control. Ideally this should be play—something physical that feels like fun and games to your child.

11. Don't be afraid to say, "You're NOT hungry! Honey, you just finished a big meal; the kitchen is closed." They are probably bored, not hungry. Shoo them outside to play or offer them a glass of water.

12. Use the Healthy Plate guidelines, page 86, and adjust the portion size for your child. Starch should be a whole grain, not more than a half a cup per meal.

13. We make sure everyone we love is getting their omega-3 and vitamin D. Recent scientific research indicates that most kids over 100 pounds need about 2,000 IU of oral vitamin D_3 daily. Yes, that's the same amount we recommended earlier for adults. We give our children (ages 13 to 26) 2,000 IU of vitamin D_3 along with about 100 percent of the daily value for other essential nutrients. We also give them 2 or 3 capsules of a highly purified omega-3 supplement each day.

CHAPTER 18

Becoming Healthy and Attractive from the Inside Out

"The artist is nothing without the gift, but the gift is nothing without the work."
–Georgia O'Keeffe

You're So Vain . . . and That's Okay!

Helena Rubinstein, in 1923, was famously quoted as saying, "There are no ugly women, only lazy ones." I know my grandmothers were operating under that truism when they were working hard to be beautiful 20-somethings in the roaring '20s. They probably followed the tried and true recipe for robust health and natural beauty: attention to detail in their personal hygiene and appearance, a diet of fresh, wholesome foods, an enthusiastic attitude, a physically active lifestyle, and plenty of rest. Yet, creating health and beauty within yourself is much more achievable today, when we have the phenomenal advantages of modern science.

I am sometimes disappointed by how little progress some individuals make, even after we spell out exactly what they need to do in order to improve their cardiovascular health, or get their diabetes under control, or lower blood pressure naturally. On the other hand, many people will jump at a chance to look more

attractive and appear younger, particularly if it's a passive interven-
tion that doesn't require any effort on their part. For instance,
liposuction is 1 of the most common surgical procedures done in
America, yet it does nothing to improve health. By contrast, if you
burn off belly fat the old-fashioned way (see Chapter 12: "Burning Off Belly Fat") you will not only feel and look better, but you
will grow much healthier too. You are going to have to get over
the passive approach if you want to thrive to your full potential. So
what can you do to look better, that just coincidentally happens to
also give you longevity with vitality?

Get a golden glow from the inside out by consuming lots
of plant-based pigments from natural, deeply-hued vegetables,
fruits, and beverages. Forget the spray tans, and definitely avoid
the tanning booths; getting color from your diet is 1 of the best
ways to look vibrant and youthful, and grow healthier at the same
time. Scientifically valid studies have consistently found that people
perceive the skin-glow that comes from a high intake of plant-
based pigments as a sign of health and vigor—even more so than
a suntan. So for each meal, consume 2 or more colors, like carrots,
tomatoes, red and orange bell peppers, darkly-colored berries
including blueberries and blackberries, and drink low-sodium V8®
juice and 1 glass of red wine daily.

Improve your posture. I try to frequently remind myself of
this, and I must admit, I tend to nag my children about posture. I will
whisper to Kathleen, my 16 year old, "Stand up straight," while we
are in church, or urge 13 year old Caroline to, "Keep your shoulders
back," as she is typing on a computer. And even though my kids ac-
cuse me of quoting imaginary scientific studies to validate my points,
a growing consensus from a wide variety of health professionals
backs me up on this issue: good posture matters a great deal—and
may even promote health and longevity. Good posture influences
not only how others perceive us, but also alters our own self-image.
A study highlighted in the January 15, 2011, issue of the *Economist*
magazine, found that practicing good posture sends a clear

message of empowerment to your inner self and helps to give you a sense that you can control your own destiny. So when you hold your head up high, pull your shoulders back, and stand erect, you not only command the respect of others, but subconsciously, you may also improve your self-esteem and self-respect. And, an improved self-image often translates into a more conscientious attitude about eating right, getting daily exercise, avoiding abuse of alcohol, drugs, and tobacco, and taking good care of yourself in general.

Still not convinced sleep is that critical? Here is more proof that you need to get 7½ to 9 hours of sleep each 24-hour cycle. The notion of beauty sleep now has science to back it up. Swedish researchers, publishing in the *British Medical Journal*, used rigorous testing to determine that "Sleep deprived people are perceived as less attractive, less healthy, and more tired compared with when they are well rested." Shocking discovery! One more reason to get to bed!

Keep your hormones, like thyroid hormone, testosterone, estrogen, growth hormone, cortisol, and insulin in their ideal ranges. This can entail many complex issues and you will almost certainly need to work with your health care providers on this one. Include these tests in your annual exam. Hormones can be regulated by diet, exercise, lifestyle changes such as sleep, and pharmaceutical or natural replacement therapies. Here's a do-it-yourself approach to staying young and strong by getting your critically important hormones into their ideal ranges: regular sexual activity with a partner—estrogen and oxytocin; weight lifting—testosterone; high intensity interval training and adequate sleep—growth hormone; meditation and prayer—cortisol; Forever Young Diet—insulin; daily aerobic exercise—adrenalin.

No added sugar! Joan avoids sweets like the plague. Sugar, like smoking, causes inflammation, which among other things causes skin wrinkles. Joan has many clients who know exactly how much sugar they can eat yet still maintain their weight in an ideal range. But even though a diet like that may not make them fat, it will promote facial wrinkles. Sugar and other easily digested carbs (like starches, breads, pasta, potatoes) cause spikes of sugar and triglycerides in the bloodstream, which in turn trigger inflammation—resulting in wrinkles, among other more potentially serious health issues.

Eat some healthy fats, preferably with each of your 3 daily meals. Extra virgin olive oil, avocados, raw or lightly salted nuts (not peanuts), and oily fish (and/or fish oil) are the best sources of healthy fats. This is great for keeping your complexion youthful and your tummy flat.

Exercise daily for 30 to 50 minutes, but avoid exhaustive, extreme exercise like running marathons or ultra-marathons. Make sure to include cardio, strength training, and stretching activities. Have a strict cutoff of 2 hours a day maximum of sitting in front of a screen during leisure time. Use some of that freed-up leisure time to invest in your romance and love life—safe sex is great for improving the quality of your life as well as your health!

Maintain a beautiful smile. A healthy and beautiful mouth isn't just a vanity issue—it's essential for keeping your heart, brain, and blood vessels healthy. Gum disease and tooth loss have been strongly linked to heart attacks, diabetes, and Alzheimer's disease. Floss daily, and brush your teeth at least twice daily—ideally with an electric device such as a Sonicare toothbrush. Drinking green tea, eliminating all foods and drinks with added sugar, and avoiding starchy carbs will also keep your teeth and gums healthy.

Inner Beauty and Strength

Dan Buettner, in his fascinating and widely-acclaimed bestseller book, *The Blue Zones* (Second Edition), searches throughout the world to discover the cultures that produce the longest-lived and healthiest people, from whom he distills longevity insights. In one interview he asks a woman named Kamanda if she had a secret that allowed her to live so gracefully to age 102. She replies, "I used to be very beautiful; I had hair that came down to my waist. It took me a long time to realize that beauty is within. It comes from not worrying so much about your own problems. Sometimes you can best take care of yourself by taking care of others." Then Buettner asked "Anything else?" She replied, "Eat your vegetables, have a positive outlook, be kind to people, and smile." Later Buettner mused that this charming little centenarian was able to convey the essence of how to optimize health and achieve longevity in just 5 sentences—a feat that he felt he needed to write a 300-page book to accomplish.

CHAPTER 19

Exercise: The Fountain of Youth

Make Time for Exercise: How and Why Cardiologists Do

We like to think of life as a grand adventure that we need to train for in order to fully appreciate all of its beauty and opportunity. When one of my patients gives me the excuse that he is too busy to find time to exercise daily, I ask him, "What fits into your hectic, over-booked schedule better, exercising a half hour daily, or being dead or disabled 24 hours a day?" Indeed, we are always talking about the importance of exercise for improving health and well-being. Fitting it into our hectic daily schedules, however, is difficult for many people. The latest studies show that 2 out of 3 Americans are not regularly active—it's a major problem.

Like many of our patients, doctors are very busy people. We usually start our days before the sun comes up, and often don't get home until it is dark. Our days are typically filled with important appointments that have been booked weeks and sometimes, months in advance. Additionally, unscheduled situations arise requiring our attention throughout the day. Still, cardiologists, as a rule, tend to be pretty darned good at not just talking the talk, but also walking the walk when it comes to fitness. One of my patients, a big and burly truck driver, told me, "Doctors these days are too skinny. Why look at you Doc, I bet you wouldn't last 2 minutes in a bar fight!" Here is some advice from cardiologists who are friends and colleagues of mine about how and why they make time for their daily exercise.

Richard Moe, MD, has been exercising every morning since he was diagnosed with high blood pressure as a 21-year-old student. Dr. Moe says the chronic health problems we tend to get are often life-long issues. When his patients ask how often they have to exercise, he responds by saying, "Just on the days when you are stressed, or overweight, or obese, or have high blood pressure, or high cholesterol, or diabetes, or heart disease." For most Americans, this means we need to exercise every day. Exercise has the power to revolutionize our health and vitality like nothing else can. Many people who exercise regularly, do so first thing in the morning, even though it means rolling out of bed a bit earlier. Dr. Moe finds that an early morning workout is the only way he can predictably exercise every day. He also finds that he generally feels better during the day if he has exercised that morning.

Working out first thing in the morning assures that you will get your fitness activity done before the rest of the world wakes up and has a chance to start harassing you with obligations. As an added perk, you won't have that nagging guilt about exercising hanging over your head for the rest of the day. If you wait until after work, many people feel too tired, hungry, or emotionally exhausted to muster the energy it takes to overcome their inertia. Joan has figured out that she doesn't allow herself the luxury of her morning shower until her exercise is done.

My good friend Anthony Magalski, MD, has a daily workout that includes strength training, like pull ups and weight lifting, as well as aerobic exercise, like running or swimming. He prefers exercising after work, often at a fitness club near his home. He regularly does interval training, which involves repeated cycles of maximal effort for about 30 to 60 seconds followed by 1 or 3 minutes of recovery. One of Tony's mottos is, "When you stop doing the hard things, life doesn't get easier; the easy things just become hard." By the way, if you are thinking about doing interval training, you may want to clear it with your physician.

What if you can't seem to drag yourself out of bed in the morning to exercise, and find you're too tired to get it done after work? A refreshing exercise session over the lunch hour just may be your ticket to fitness. Get out for a 15 to 30-minute brisk walk over the noon hour, and you can still have time to eat a light and healthy lunch. Exercise in the middle of the day is not just convenient, but also invigorating. Studies show that a 30 to 40 minute workout at lunchtime lowers stress, improves productivity, and leaves you happier for the rest of the day. I personally find this to be one of my favorite times to exercise, and I do it whenever I get the chance. Sometimes, I start my afternoon schedule a little flushed and sweaty but my patients just laugh when I explain that I just came back from my mid-day workout.

I also often exercise after work, and indeed science shows that the late afternoon is predictably the time of the day when your body is most ready for exercise, even if your mind might not be. Your muscles are stretched out, your fuel tank is full, and your hormones are in their ideal ranges for physical exertion. My friend Bob shuns morning workouts, but has developed a habit of mid- to late-afternoon exercise. Even when he comes home from work feeling unmotivated or fatigued, he has learned to force himself to work out. "After the first several minutes of forced exercise I discover renewed energy and vitality. I finish the workout with zeal, and it wakes me up, shakes off my lethargy and allows me to be more productive and enthused for the rest of the evening. I find that the older I get, the more important this exercise-induced energy boost becomes," he told me.

Organic Fitness: Back to the Future

From the inception of the human genus, homo, approximately 2.4 million years ago, our ancestors lived as hunter-gatherers for approximately 84,000 generations. Survival in the hunter-gatherer mode of life required a large amount of daily energy expenditure in activities such as food and water procurement, social interaction, escape from predators, maintenance of shelter, and clothing. This lifestyle represents the exercise patterns for which we remain genetically adapted even today. Dramatic improvements in technology over the past few generations have made our lives ever more convenient but in so doing, have markedly reduced the amount of physical work required in our daily lives.

Especially in recent years, technological advances have in many cases completely eliminated the need for physical activity in our day-to-day routines. I often ask my patients if they have chest pain or shortness of breath when they exert themselves, and they often reply, "I am not sure; I never exert myself." For hunter-gatherers exercise was not optional. Their harsh world required daily physical labor for nearly their entire life. An adult hunter-gatherer would not consider setting off on a run for recreation or repeatedly lifting a heavy stone simply to improve their fitness level. To the contrary, natural selection endowed them with an instinct compelling them to 'move when you have to, and rest when you can.' Many of their waking hours were necessarily consumed with the physical activities demanded of everyday life.

Retirement was not an option for hunter-gatherers. Their activities of daily life were all the exercise that Stone Age people would have ever needed to maintain superb general fitness. Instincts to preserve energy and strength conferred survival advantages to hunter-gatherers. These instincts, still apparent in modern humans, are now harmful in the sedentary over-fed 21st century milieu in which we live. Our inborn proclivity to take the path of least resistance while living and working in our ultra-convenient, highly-mechanized environment plays a major role in the health woes plaguing modern Americans.

Achieving Hunter-Gatherer Vitality and Strength in the 21st Century

The prescription of physical activities listed below is the closest thing you and I will ever have to a cure-all wonder drug. These are the types of daily activities that were required of our ancient ancestors. By incorporating these kinds of exercises into your daily routine, you will be fulfilling your genetic destiny, which will allow you to realize the awesome potential for vitality, resilience, and strength that nature has encoded within your genome.

A large amount of light to moderate activity such as walking was required. Hard days were typically followed by an easy day, but every day a variety of physical activities had to be accomplished just to provide for the basic human needs. The hunter-gatherers typically burned at least 600 to 1,000 calories daily with exercise alone, about 3 times what the average American adult burns.

Cross-training is essential and should include exercises focusing on strength-building and endurance and flexibility. Walking was often done while carrying weight loads such as children, water, food, wood, stones, etc. The lack of this regular lifting and carrying likely accounts in part for the common occurrence of osteoporosis (weakening of the bones) today. Look for opportunities to carry things.

In general, hunter-gatherers were virtually never overweight or obese, which reduced trauma to their joints. They were barefoot or wore simple sandals. The use of expensive, heavily cushioned running shoes with elevated heels and excessive anti-pronation stability control may actually increase problems with plantar fasciitis, hamstring injuries, and Achilles' tendonitis. Wear simpler, less padded running or walking shoes, and when you can, opt for softer and more forgiving natural surface like dirt, grass, bark, or gravel paths (avoid concrete and asphalt surfaces when possible).

Virtually all of the exercise was done outdoors in the natural world. Outdoor activities improve mood, provide opportunities to get some sunlight so as to keep your vitamin D levels up, and make it easier for most people to stick with regular exercise program for the long-term. Our ancestors did most of their physical exercise in social settings, usually small bands of individuals who were hunting, gathering, or working together on various chores. Even today we find that people who exercise with other people tend to be more enthusiastic and consistent about getting regular exercise. Find your tribe!

It's no coincidence that dogs and humans are such good friends: genetic evidence suggests that our 2 species have been co-evolving for as long as 135,000 years—back when our ancestors weren't fully human yet and our canine companions were still wolves. This cooperation improved the hunting success, protection from predators, and chances for survival for both of the early humans and the tame wolves. In other words, dogs and humans appear to be genetically designed by nature to be outdoor exercise companions. Indeed, you may have noticed that generally most of the people who are outside exercising during unpleasant weather tend be folks like me, whose dogs coaxed them outdoors for some fresh air. My dogs are always available and enthusiastic when it comes to outdoor play, and to me that makes them wonderful exercise partners.

Our ancestors regularly engaged in ceremonial and celebratory dancing, sometimes for up to 1 or 2 hours. Dancing can be a cool and hip form of exercise that improves fitness and reduces stress.

Except for the very young and the very old, all individuals were, by necessity, physically active almost their entire lives. Even so, ample time for rest, relaxation, and sleep was generally available to ensure complete recovery after strenuous exertion.

Hunter Gatherer Activity	Modern Equivalent Activity	Calories Burned per Hour of Activity
Carrying logs	Carrying groceries, luggage	800
Running (cross country)	Running (cross country)	700
Carrying meat (20kg) back to camp	Wearing backpack while walking	650
Carrying young child	Carrying young child	600
Hunting, stalking animals	Interval training	550
Digging	Gardening	530
Dancing (ceremonial)	Dancing (vigorous)	400
Carrying, stacking rock	Lifting weights	400
Butchering large animal	Splitting wood with axe	360
Walking – normal pace (fields and hills)	Walking – brisk pace	350
Gathering plant foods	Weeding garden	300
Shelter construction	Carpentry, general	200
Tool construction	Vigorous housework	200

What Have You Done for Me Lately?

Sometimes when I ask my patients "What do you do for exercise," I hear in reply, "I was a varsity swimmer in college." Now, impressive as that may be, it's completely irrelevant to his or her current health status. Darwin's radical 'survival of the fittest' concept is true today as it was for our stone-age ancestors. What you did decades ago or even last year doesn't matter. Your body and brain want to know, "What have you done for me lately?"

A study of over 6,000 people followed for 6 years found that next to age, fitness, measured simply by how many minutes a person could exercise on a treadmill test, was the strongest predictor of survival. The fitness level was more important that their blood pressure, cholesterol, family history, or even whether or not they smoked. And fitness is an easily modifiable risk factor—simply get out there and do something physically demanding on a daily basis.

The obligations and stress of our busy world make it difficult to keep up the incentive for exercise; so rely on structure in your life more than willpower. Carve out time in your day for exercise, ideally first thing in the morning. Make it protected time for you and fiercely guard it. When I roll out of bed each morning to go for a run, a bike ride, or a swim, I often don't really feel like exercising. But I do it because it's just a habit. If I don't, Joan notices that our 2 border collies and I are much more difficult to live with. After about the first 5 minutes, I can feel my engines firing up and I'm happy to be out there. Even though you may not feel like exercising when you first wake up in the morning, once you begin your workout it will become second nature. The rest of the day you will be happier, healthier, more focused, efficient, and productive.

> "Walking is the best possible exercise.
> Habituate yourself to walking outdoors."
> –Thomas Jefferson

Catch the Heel-Toe Express

We are not so much *born to run*, as we are *born to walk*. Our pre-human ancestors first stood upright and began to walk about 2.5 million years ago. Since then, nature has shaped our bodies to be highly efficient walking creatures. As humans came to inhabit every corner of our world by walking across, over, and around the earth. Only 150 years ago, 90 percent of the world's population lived out in the natural world or on farms. Like our ancient forebears, these people walked while they built their homes and cleared their land. They walked as they planted, tended, and harvested their crops and carried babies and water. They walked as they gathered plants and stalked game. They spent much of their waking time walking, often as they even socialized with family and friends.

A scientific consensus is building that emphasizes cumulative daily walking. Studies show that walking during the course of your daily activity can improve your health as well or better than daily workouts in a fitness facility. The health benefits associated with walking include lower risks for high blood pressure, diabetes, obesity, cardiovascular disease, joint disease, depression, anxiety, and early death. The bottom line is simply that regular walking throughout the day will improve your health. On the flip side, inactivity, or being sedentary, leads to poor health, obesity, disability, and premature death.

Certainly, high-intensity interval training, and weight training to build strength provide benefits even above and beyond those noted from just walking. However, the average American is either not interested in, or not capable of, performing a strenuous, heart-pounding workout that leaves him or her sweaty and breath-less. On the other hand, a great deal of low to moderate inten-sity physical activity can provide most of the physical and mental benefits of a high-intensity program, but it requires more of a time commitment.

Are you looking for a way to save time while getting fit? When I round on my hospital patients, I make a habit of shunning the elevators and taking the stairs instead. I tell my entourage of medical students and residents, "The stairs are quicker, and these short bouts of stair-climbing are like high-intensity intervals that we can do in between seeing our patients." I often wear a high-tech pedometer called Fitbit which tracks each day the number of steps taken, miles covered, calories burned, stairs climbed, and also tracks time slept during the night. A pedometer makes me feel like I 'get credit' for going out of my way to walk more and take the stairs every chance I get. I shoot for at least 10,000 steps per day, which is about 5 miles. To attain that goal I usually have to get out for 2 mile run or walk sometime during the day.

How to Be a Hottie—In More Ways Than One

No, this is not just your imagination playing tricks on you. Your metabolism does slow down substantially as the years roll by. So while you may have been able to inhale a half of pizza during your partying days back in college without developing a muffin-top, your body won't let you get away with that today. Most individuals gain about a pound a year as they get older, and it gets worse: they actually gain about a pound and a half of fat each year while at the same time lose a half pound of valuable muscle. And since muscle burns more calories than fat, our metabolism slows down as we age—about 3 percent per decade. By the time a woman reaches menopause her body burns about 200 fewer calories each day. Additionally, at menopause a woman's body shifts its pattern of fat storage from the hips to the abdomen, making her look and feel older, and increasing risks for diabetes and heart disease.

So how do you to keep your metabolism stoked and your home fires burning hot? Simple—add more muscle to your frame, which not only makes you sturdier, sexier, and stronger, but also cranks up your metabolic furnace so that you burn many more calories at rest. It only takes about 20 to 30 minutes of focused strength training 2 or 3 times weekly to gain about 3 pounds of muscle in 10 weeks' time—which is like turning back the metabolic clock and making you 5 years younger. This modest increase in muscle mass will burn hundreds of extra calories each day just to 'keep the furnace running and lights on.' You will also need to follow the diet in this book. This combination of muscle-building exercise and an ideal diet will give you a youthful waist, better posture, and a shapely bootie—and keep you hot and sexy-looking.

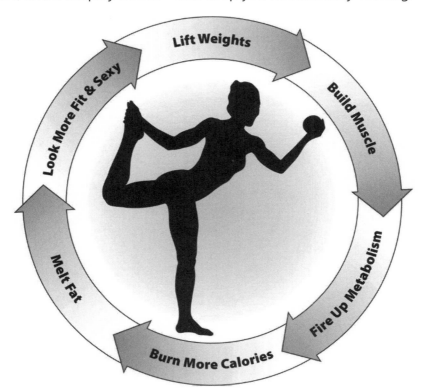

Build a Whole New You with Strength Training

Weight lifting can be simple. Start with a weight that you can lift at least 5 times (reps) but not more than about 10 or 15 reps before your muscles fatigue to the point of being unable to do even 1 more rep. Do at least 2 or 3 sets of several different strength-training exercises (lifts). Good old-fashioned push-ups are also a great strength-training exercise you can do almost any-where, or anytime—believe me, I have done push-ups everywhere from beaches to airports to hotel rooftops.

When starting a weight lifting regimen, it's a great idea to work with an experienced trainer so that you know the proper form and don't overdo it at first and injure yourself. Squats, lunges, dead lifts, arm curls, and straight-arm dumbbell raises are among the most effective weight lifting exercises. Be careful about lift-ing weights over your head—this can put excessive stress on the shoulders, and predispose to torn rotator cuff muscles—an ex-tremely common injury that often requires surgery. Finally, make sure you are eating enough protein, and taking your vitamin D and omega-3. These steps will help you to build muscle and bone and speed your recovery after a workout.

CHAPTER 20

Run For Your Life ...
at a Comfortable Pace, Not Too Far

"Life is short. Don't run so fast you miss it."
–Raffaella Monne (a 107-year-old woman from Sardinia)

The Dangers of Excessive Exercise

During the Greco-Persian War in 490 BCE, Phidippides, a 40-year-old herald messenger (professional running-courier), ran the 26 miles from a battlefield near Marathon, Greece, into Athens carrying momentous news of Greek victory. Upon arriving at the Acropolis he proclaimed, "Joy, we have won!" He then immediately collapsed and died. Fast-forward about 2,500 years to an era when the baby-boomers came of age and the sport of long distance running boomed. The prevailing logic held that aerobic exercise is clearly good for one's health and that if some is good, more must be better. In 1975, Dr. Thomas Bassler, a physician-runner, boldly proclaimed that if you could run a marathon you were immune to coronary heart disease death. This urban myth has been long-since disproven; indeed an emerging body of evidence suggests the opposite: extreme endurance exercise may exact a toll on cardio-vascular health.

"Show Me the Bodies"

After our recent articles on this topic, Amby Burfoot, winner of the 1968 Boston Marathon and Editor-at-Large for *Runner's World* magazine, challenged our assertions about the dangers of extreme endurance efforts by demanding, "Show me the bodies." Amby has a good point; the risk of dropping dead in a marathon is remote, about 1 in 100,000 participants. But the occasional marathoner or triathlete who dies while strenuously exercising is the 'canary in the coal mine.' Chronic extreme exercise appears to cause excessive wear-and-tear on the heart, inducing adverse changes in the heart's structure and making it irritable and prone to dangerous rhythms. These abnormalities offset some of the cardiac benefits and longevity improvements bestowed by moderate physical activity. Thus, even though chronic extreme exercise may not kill you, it might erase many of the health advantages of regular moderate exercise.

In fact, developing a routine that includes moderate to strenuous exercise is probably the single best step a person can take to ensure robust cardiac health. In a study of 416,000 adults followed for a mean of 8 years, 40 to 50 minutes per day of vigorous exercise reduced risk of death by about 40 percent. In that study, at about 45 minutes a point of diminishing returns was reached whereby longer exercise efforts did not appear to translate into lower death risk. Light to moderate physical activity reduced death rates too, albeit not as strongly; but in this case more physical activity appeared to be better with no plateau out to 110 minutes daily.

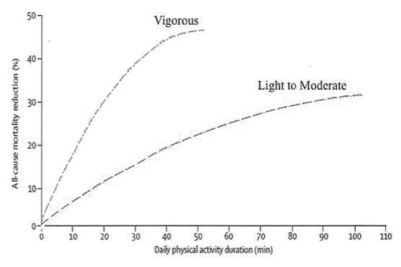

Source: *Lancet*. Exercise and life expectancy. Letter to the editor. 379:799.2012

Indeed, if we had a pill that confers all the benefits of exercise, many physicians might be out looking for work. Approximately 30 to 45 minutes of daily vigorous exercise significantly reduces risks for many maladies including: early death, Alzheimer's Disease, heart attack, diabetes, osteoporosis, and depression. Yet, as can be expected with any potent drug, an insufficient dose will not bestow the optimal benefits, while an excessive dose can cause harm, and even death in extreme overdoses.

The survival-of-the-fittest notion does not fully apply to the modern world, where it appears that even the moderately fit tend to have excellent cardiovascular health and remarkable longevity. Studies of fitness, as measured by peak performance on a treadmill, show a curvilinear relationship whereby improvements from unfit to moderately fit confer dramatic reductions in morbidity and mortality. However, improving one's fitness level from very good to exceptional does not seem to translate into additional gains in cardiovascular durability and life expectancy. To put it another way, if one is training to be able to run at speeds above 7.5 miles per hour it is for some reason other than further improvements in cardiac health and longevity.

Cardiovascular Damage from Excessive Exercise

High-intensity exercise sessions lasting beyond 1 to 2 hours can over-tax your heart with too much work and pumping of blood, eventually overstretching the heart and ripping apart some of its muscle cells. Although within 1 week these transitory abnormalities usually return to baseline, after years to decades of excessive exercise and repetitive injury this pattern can lead to patchy scarring in the pliable walls of the heart. Additionally, long-term excessive exercise may accelerate aging in the heart as evidenced by an increase in the calcium deposition and plaque formation in the walls of the coronary arteries, and stiffening of the heart and major blood vessels.

At rest the heart pumps about 5 quarts per minute; with strenuous aerobic exercise the cardiac output can rise up to 5 to 7-fold, pumping up to 25 to 35 quarts per minute. This massive increase in cardiac work is what the heart is designed to do for short bursts, or even for up to as long as 30 or 50 minutes continuously. However, with long, hard, and continuous efforts, these high volumes can over-stretch the chambers, eventually disrupting cardiac muscle fibers. The presence of sustained exercise-induced elevations in adrenalin and pro-oxidant free radicals worsen the situation by adding inflammation to the injury, leading eventually to fibrosis and stiffening of the cardiovascular structures.

Cardiologists from Minnesota evaluated a group of runners who had completed at least 25 marathons over 25 years and found a 60 percent increase in coronary plaque burden in the walls of their heart arteries compared to non-exercisers of a similar age. These findings were replicated by a group from Germany who showed increased coronary artery plaque in 108 chronic marathoners compared to inactive controls. This scarring can set the stage for dangerous heart rhythms, such as atrial fibrillation, which is increased by approximately 5-fold in veteran endurance athletes.

An enlightening study by Benito reinforced the concept of cardiac damage from chronic excessive exercise. Mice after being forced to run to exhaustion every day for 4 months showed the same cardiac enlargement, scarring and predisposition to dangerous heart rhythms that have been documented in some veteran extreme endurance athletes. Encouragingly, when the mice were withdrawn from the "Iron-Mouse" training regimen and allowed to resume normal mouse physical activity levels their cardiac abnormalities showed marked improvements, even showing regression of scarring in the heart muscle and resolution of the tendency toward dangerous heart rhythms.

Phidippides Cardiomyopathy

Born to Run is a nonfiction bestseller book published in 2009 that glamorizes ultra-endurance running. The story's hero is Micah True, an American who dropped out of modern civilization to live and run with the Tarahumara Indians in Mexico. Nicknamed Caballo Blanco, or white horse for his legendary running endurance, he routinely ran daily distances 10 to 100 miles. On March 27, 2012, while out on a routine 12-mile training run in New Mexico, Micah True dropped dead at age 58. On autopsy his heart was enlarged and thickened, with inflammation and fibrotic scarring. The coroner classified his death as likely due to a lethal rhythm abnormality caused by a weak and diseased heart. When considered in the context of True's decades-long lifestyle of daily ultra-endurance running, we suspect that the autopsy findings were an example of Phidippides Cardiomyopathy: the constellation of cardiac pathology that has been in the observed in hearts of some veteran extreme endurance athletes.

Moderate Exercise: the Sweet-spot for Longevity

Two very recent studies may revolutionize our thinking about running and its health effects. One followed 52,000 people for up to 3 decades, and showed that the 14,000 runners in that study had a significantly lower risk of death compared with the 42,000 non-runners. Yet, when they sub-grouped the runners by weekly mileage, those who ran over 20 or 25 miles per week seemed to lose their survival advantage over the non-runners (see figure). On the other hand, those who ran between 5 and 20 miles total per week enjoyed a 25 percent decrease in risk of death during follow up. The same pattern emerged for speed of running: the fast runners, those running typically over 8 miles an hour, appeared to get no mortality benefit compared to the non-runners; while those who fared best usually ran about 6 to 7 miles per hour—a comfortable jog for most people. Additionally, the individuals who ran 6 or 7 days per week appeared to lose the mortality benefits; whereas the survival advantages accrued best for those who ran 2 to 5 days per week.

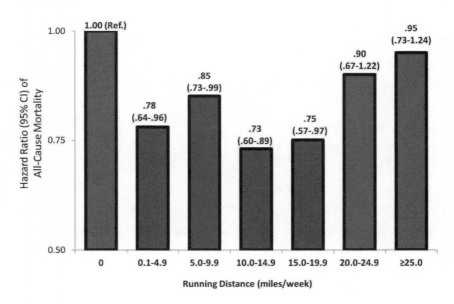

Source: O'Keefe, *Mayo Clinic Proceedings*, 87(11):1133-1134. Nov 2012

The Copenhagen City Heart Study showed remarkably similar results. After following 20,000 Danes since 1976 they found that the joggers lived about 6 years longer than the non-runners, with a 44 percent lower risk of death during the study. Intriguingly, those who did best were the people who jogged at a slow-to-average pace, for 1 to 2.5 hours per week total, accumulated during 2 or 3 sessions. According to Dr. Peter Schnohr, the study's director, "The relationship appears much like alcohol intakes—mortality is lower in people reporting moderate jogging than in non-joggers or those undertaking extreme levels of exercise."

The U-Curve of Exercise

Hippocrates, the father of medicine, and a contemporary of Phidippides in ancient Greece, taught, "The right amount of nourishment and exercise, not too much, not too little, is the safest way to health." If you listen to your body this is just common sense. Yet, nothing we have published previously has stirred so much controversy, especially among the general public. Increasingly our culture is one of extremes: during the past 30 years, obesity has tripled in the United States, while during the same time the number of people completing a marathon has risen 20-fold. On one side of the U-curve, the couch loungers/channel surfers embrace this message as justification for continuing their sedentary lifestyle. And, on the far end of the U-curve, the extreme exercise aficionados want to ignore the message and instead kill the messenger. As with many things in life, the safe and comfortable zone at the bottom of the U curve— moderate exercise—is the sweet-spot for which we should try to aim.

So while it's true that exercise confers powerful health benefits, the common belief that more is better is clearly not true. The unique and potent benefits of exercise are best bestowed by moderate physical activity. The exercise patterns for maximizing cardiovascular fitness/peak aerobic capacity are very different from those that promote ideal health, durability and overall longevity. Stated another way, if your goal in life is to compete in the marathon or triathlon of the Rio de Janeiro Olympics in 2016, you will need to do high intensity exercise for hours each day. But, for those whose goal is to be alive and well while watching the 2052 Olympics from the stands, then exercise and physical activity at lower intensities and durations would be more ideal.

Take-Home Message

Limit your vigorous exercise to about 30 to 50 minutes per day. If you really want to do a marathon or full distance triathlon, or some other extreme endurance event do just 1 or a few, cross it off your bucket list, and then settle into safer and healthier exercise patterns. On the other hand, light or moderate intensity exercise does not cause the dose-dependent cardiac overuse injury associated with excessive endurance exercise. A routine of moderate physical activity will add life to your years, as well as years to your life. In contrast, running too fast, too far, and for too many years may speed one's progress towards the finish line of life.

Avoiding Exercise-Induced Cardiovascular Damage

Suggestions for an exercise routine that will optimize heath, fitness and longevity without causing damage to the heart and blood vessels and predisposing to dangerous rhythms:

- Avoid a daily routine of exhaustive strenuous exercise for periods greater than 1 hour continuously. An ideal target might be not more than 7 hours weekly of cumulative strenuous endurance exercise.

- When doing exhaustive aerobic exercise, take intermittent rest periods, even for a few minutes at an easier pace, such slowing down to walk in the middle of a run.

- Accumulate a large amount (shoot for at least 3 to 5 hours weekly) of low intensity cardio activity, such as walking, gardening, housekeeping, etc. Avoid prolonged sitting. Walk intermittently throughout the day. Look for opportunities to take the stairs.

- Once or twice weekly for 15 to 30 minutes perform high-intensity interval training such as Cross-Fit. This is more effective in improving overall fitness and peak aerobic capacity than is continuous aerobic exercise, despite a much shorter total accumulated exercise time spent doing the interval workout.

- Incorporate cross training using stretching, yoga for example, and strength training into the weekly exercise routine. This confers multi-faceted fitness and reduces the burden of cardiac work compared to a routine of daily long-distance endurance training.

- Avoid chronically competing in very long distance races, such as marathons, ultra-marathons, Iron-man distance triathlons, 100-mile bicycle races, etc., especially after age 45 or 50.

- Individuals over 45 or 50 years of age should reduce the intensity and durations of endurance exercise training sessions, and allow more recovery time.

Keeping Your Muscles and Joints Healthy

It is much easier to maintain an active lifestyle and a dynamic and strong heart if your joints and muscles stay healthy. However, sore muscles and aching joints are among the most common complaints we hear from our friends and patients. Most people resort to prescription pain relievers, or high doses of agents such as ibuprofen or naproxen; all of which just mask the pain and can be dangerous.

Instead, we suggest that you concentrate on using a natural approach to make your musculoskeletal system healthier. When walking or running, try to choose softer surfaces such as dirt, grass or gravel. Additionally, try to include some non-jarring aerobic exercises such as swimming, cycling, or gliding on an elliptical trainer. Incorporating strength training (such as weight lifting) and stretching (such as yoga) into your weekly routine will also help to keep your muscles and joints strong and supple.

Safe and effective natural supplements can also improve vigor and resiliency of your joints and muscles. Omega-3 will improve post-exercise muscle inflammation and soreness and also reduces joint soreness. SAMe, and/or Glucosamine/Chondroitin can also help some people with sore joints. If you have low vitamin D levels, getting your level back into the normal range (at least 30 ng/ml) will help to reduce joint and muscle inflammation, strengthen muscles and bones, and reduce musculoskeletal pain. Finally, Coenzyme Q-10 is a very important compound naturally found in high levels in healthy youthful muscles. Supplementing with Coenzyme Q-10 150 to 400 mg daily will often markedly improve muscular soreness, especially if you are taking a statin cholesterol-lowering drug. The average American adult is deficient in these important and natural compounds and supplementing these levels back into the ideal ranges will often lessen the pain, and also improve the health of the joints and muscles.

CHAPTER 21

A Good Night's Sleep: Make This Luxury a Top Priority

*"A good laugh and a long sleep are
the best cures in a doctor's book."*
–Irish Proverb

As I always do with my patients, I asked Ray if he snores while he sleeps. His wife, Laura, chimed in, "Yes, he snores very loudly!" Ray protested, "I sleep like a baby, and I never hear myself snoring. Besides, Laura sleeps in a different bedroom at the other end of the house, so how would she know?" Laura responded, "You sleep like a baby all right—every 2 hours you wake up cranky, and have to pee and eat before you go back to sleep."

You think time spent sleeping is wasted time? Think again. Throughout the course of a typical rush-rush, harried, and hectic day your body and your mind are constantly barraged by a variety of stresses. By the time you finally flick off the lights, slide under the cool smooth sheets, and drift off into dreamland, you are desperately in need of a long and peaceful sleep. Your muscles relax, your brain waves slow and synchronize, your breathing becomes slow and deep, your blood pressure and pulse settle into nice, low-normal levels, your stress hormones plummet, and the NK (Natural Killer) cells of your immune system kick into high gear eradicating any foreign enemies like cancer cells, bacteria, and viruses that are constantly trying to invade your system. Nothing will rejuvenate and revitalize your brain and your body like a great night's sleep.

Modern life is too often full of pressures, anxieties, and hassles and this causes our flight-or-fight hormones like adrenalin (epinephrine) and cortisol to rise. These stress hormones raise your levels of blood pressure, glucose, and cholesterol and trigger cravings, especially for junk food. If you short-change your sleep, these stress hormones escalate and can over time lead to obesity and many diseases. Deep and restful sleep calms your system, and re-sets these stress hormones back down to their healthy ranges; and you awaken renewed, recharged, and reinvigorated. Problems that felt overwhelming when you collapsed into bed just 8 hours before often seem perfectly manageable in the bright light of a new day when you feel rested and re-energized.

A team of West Virginia University researchers analyzed data from more than 30,000 adults, and found that the amount of time during each 24-hour day you routinely spend sleeping has a powerful effect on your risk of suffering a cardiovascular catas-trophe such as heart attack or stroke. Sleeping less than 7 hours a day, including naps, can double or triple your risk of heart attack or stroke, compared to people who sleep 7 to 8 hours a day. But, be-fore you sleepy heads get too smug, remember, all things in mod-eration. It turns out that sleeping over 9 hours on a routine basis, is also linked to increased risk of cardiovascular disease compared to those people who routinely sleep 7½ to 9 hours.

"When I die, I would rather go peacefully, just drifting off to sleep like my grandfather did; not screaming in terror like the passengers in his car."
–Jack Handey

Too little sleep can lead to motor vehicle accidents, high blood pressure, pre-diabetes and diabetes, dangerous heart rhythms, and elevated stress hormones. Yet, our favorite reason to get 7½ to 9 hours of sleep nightly is simply to feel happier and more productive. Joan and I find that it's difficult to really feel enthused, optimistic, and energetic when we haven't had enough sleep. In our opinion, a restful night's sleep is one of life's exquisite and under-rated pleasures. Too many of us get distracted by TV, computers, movies, work, and cell phones and skimp on time spent sleeping. Make it a priority to get 7½ to 9 hours of sleep each 24-hour period. A good night's sleep exerts profound benefits on the brain: sharper concentration, happier mood, better short-term memory, improved productivity, and enhanced creativity.

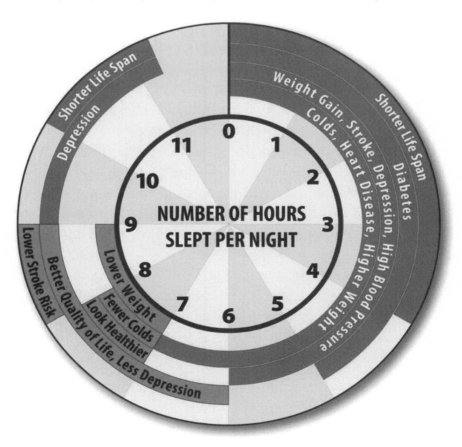

How to Sleep Like a Kitten

Keep your bedroom dark, cool, and quiet; and reserve your bed almost exclusively for sleep and sex. Make it a point to not watch TV or use your computer in bed. These kind of bedtime habits can interfere with your ability to sleep soundly. On the other hand, many people find it relaxing and even conducive to restful sleep to read quietly in bed before turning out the lights and snuggling in for the night. Remember to avoid heavily caffeinated beverages after about 2:00 or 3:00 p.m., because caffeine takes up to 24 hours to be fully eliminated from your system and is a very common and often overlooked cause of difficulty falling and staying asleep at night.

A low-dose aspirin (81 mg) is a surprisingly good sleep aid, and when taken at bedtime, will gently lower your blood pressure during the night. Another safe, natural, non-habit-forming and effective sleep aid is sustained-release melatonin, 3 mg, which can be taken alone or with the low-dose aspirin at bedtime. Many people use products like Tylenol PM, which contain Benadryl and acetaminophen. These are modestly effective and non-habit-forming sleep aids, but they tend to dry out your mucosal surfaces in the mouth and throat, and the latest data show that they also can predispose to weight gain. Prescription sleep aids like Ambien and Temazepam are very effective in the short term, but are extremely habit-forming. They are okay for unusual circumstances (for example, the night before a big occasion, or in the midst of a very stressful time of your life), but if you take them more than once or twice a week, you will likely become addicted to the point where you won't be able to fall asleep without them. We have many patients who have been taking Ambien every single night for over a decade because when they don't take it, they can't fall asleep.

Avoid drinking alcohol within 4 hours of bedtime. Although you might drift off easier after 1 or more drinks, the alcohol in your bloodstream will prevent you from obtaining restful and restorative sleep and will worsen any tendency to snore. Even if you are emotionally exhausted, you may have a difficult time falling and staying asleep if you haven't had enough physical activity during the day. One of the best ways to improve your quality of sleep is to get 30 to 60 minutes of moderate or vigorous exercise each day. Follow these suggestions, and not only will you get the sleep your body needs, you'll reduce your risk for heart attack and stroke.

Your kindergarten teacher was on to something when she insisted that you curl up for an afternoon nap. A study of 23,000 Greek adults showed that occasionally napping decreased one's risk for coronary heart disease by 12 percent, and regular napping (defined as laying down during the day to rest for about 30 minutes at least 3 times weekly) slashed the risk by a remarkable 37 percent. Napping lowers stress hormones and gives your mind, body and heart a respite from the day's pressures. I try to nap for 30 minutes on Saturday and Sunday and when on vacation. Joan is devoted napster—she curls up almost every afternoon for a catnap—about 20 to 30 minutes when possible. However, when her schedule is especially overbooked, even a short 5 or 10 minute power-nap can make Joan a happy camper again.

CHAPTER 22

Love and Survival

The Brain-Heart Connection

Your thoughts powerfully influence your heart. In a paper entitled "Behavioral Cardiology" published in the *Journal of Preventive Cardiology*, we outlined how chronic thoughts can crystallize into reality by altering human biology. When emotions like enthusiasm, optimism, kindness, happiness, love, and gratitude regularly flow through your consciousness they will send rejuvenation and healing signals to every cell in your body. As great as it is to be on the receiving end of those emotions, it is even better for your heart, brain, and body to be the one showing kindness to others, conveying love, feeling gratitude for your blessings, and looking to the future with enthusiasm and hope. Attributes like passion for a cause, a positive outlook, and a sense of humor seem to promote contentment, resilience, longevity, and vigor.

In contrast, the toxic effects of negative emotions cast a shadow of darkness over the mind-heart connection. Of all the emotions, hopelessness stands out as the most lethal to your health. Each morning when the sun dawns, greet it with gratitude and hope; trust that the new day is an opportunity for a fresh start.

A Yale study by Becca Levy, PhD, reported that older men and women with a positive attitude enjoyed a 7-year survival advantage compared to their more negative contemporaries. Maggie is a lovely and energetic woman who suffered a heart attack 7 years ago. She was getting along famously well until she noticed worsening shortness of breath and fatigue. Rather than dismissing it as old age she surmised that it might be a sign of a recurring heart problem. Indeed, her angiogram showed a very severe blockage in the left main coronary artery—a life threatening problem. I explained that coronary bypass surgery is the treatment of choice for left main disease; but that at age 90, it would understandable if she wanted to forgo this highly invasive approach and instead just hope for the best with medications. She asked, "Will this surgery fix my heart so I can get back to a full life again?" I replied, "It would be your best shot at it, but there is no guarantee." She said, "Well, Dr. O'Keefe, I have a lot of things I want to do yet, and I know I can't get them done in the shape I'm in now. So let's get my heart fixed; what do I have to lose?" Maggie went on to have the surgery and after a speedy recovery she is now busily re-engaged in life. She has even made a bunch of new friends at her local community fitness center. Maggie's spunky, irrepressible, can-do attitude is a great example how optimism can influence longevity.

> "The meeting of 2 personalities is like the contact of 2 chemical substances; if there is any reaction, both are transformed."
> –Carl Jung

It's Not All About You

Danny is a delightful 80 year old who still works as a courier and office boy for a large bank; he brags that he is their oldest full-time employee. He also volunteers as an usher for his church, where according to him, he is always getting hit on by more than a few of the smiling and attentive widows. Danny is not someone

I would describe as a poster child for the Cardio Wellness Clinic. Despite my efforts through the years to reform his diet, he remains obese and frequently indulges his cravings for sweets. Yet he remains remarkably healthy and enthusiastic, and I am sure that Danny's continuing engagement with his community has something to do with his hale and hearty good health.

Dr. Andrew Weil writes, "Doing good for others brings a very tangible reward in the form of benefits to physical and mental health." A large study found that people who volunteer regularly are, amazingly, 10 times more likely to be in good health than those who don't volunteer. Another scientific study reported that people over age 55 who volunteer for 2 or more organizations were 44 percent less likely to die during follow up than those who didn't volunteer—a reduction in mortality as impressive as that conferred by exercising 4 times weekly, or kicking a cigarette habit for good.

Happiness Is Overrated

An emerging scientific discipline called positive psychology, finds that happiness, as usually defined—experiencing pleasure or cheerful feelings—is not nearly as important to long-term mental well-being and physical health as is the type of fulfillment and satisfaction that results from engaging in meaningful activity, like helping others, working on realizing your innate potential, or investing time and energy in a cause that inspires you. Psychology experts believe our modern American obsession with personal status and material things, and the emphasis on the relentless pursuit of happiness and immediate pleasure may be doing us more harm than good.

Not that fun and pleasure are bad things, indeed they bring one type of happiness, but not the kind of deep satisfaction that translates into a meaningful life. A deeper sense of contentment comes from making it a priority to live with a sense of purpose, while pursuing goals that bring meaning to their life. Dr. Ed Diener, an expert on positive psychology, advises, "Quit sitting around worrying about yourself and get focused on your goals."

As my wife Joan often tells our children and me, "It's not all about you." Ironically, if you worry less about what makes you happy, you tend to become happier. You are unlikely to find happiness by looking within yourself; when you shift your attention from yourself to the wider world, you will become less self-absorbed and stop ruminating. Get out there and immerse yourself in the life around you, and find a cause to which you might contribute some of your time and energy. Oliver Segovia recently wrote in the *Harvard Business Review*, "Happiness comes from the intersection of what you love, what you're good at, and what the world needs. What problems are you helping to solve?" Troubles you might be inspired to invest some of your energy into are not hard to find, whether big problems like global climate change, social injustice, the obesity epidemic, education, and poverty, or more personal concerns like problems in your family, school, church, or community. You will be more likely to be motivated by issues that you can relate to on a personal level. Try to become more aware to the problems faced by unfortunate and marginalized people. Each of us has his or her own unique talents and life circumstances along our journey. Our day-to-day struggles can bring out the best in us and define who we are. Particularly when we are experiencing tough times ourselves or see others struggling, we can find fulfillment by rolling up our sleeves, rising to the occasion and doing what we can to make a positive difference.

A Prescription for Happiness and Longevity

Andrew Weil, M.D., in his fabulous and enlightened book, *Spontaneous Happiness*, writes that the average person believes that what he or she needs to be happy is more money, or a new car, or a new lover, or something else that we yearn for, but do not have. Dr. Weil says that the actual emotional reward of getting and having things is usually much less than one imagined. Instead, his advice for emotional and physical well-being includes:

- Remind yourself to feel grateful for all that you have, and learn to express gratitude frequently to the people in your life. This single step is the best and easiest way to move your emotional set point toward greater happiness and positivity. Lately, before I drift off to sleep each night, I try to reflect upon a few of my many blessings.

- Consider adopting an animal companion. The emotional rewards of animal companionship are powerful.

- Try to be more compassionate and empathetic to the people in your world. Make it a point to put others first more often, without neglecting your own needs. One of the best ways to become happier and healthier yourself is to try to help others in need; this can also inspire you to overcome the hurdles in your own life.

- Grant forgiveness as a strategy to cleanse your mind of negative thoughts and emotions that might be interfering with your quest for ideal health. Forgiving is particularly healing for you, more so than anyone else. Harboring resentment is like swallowing a poison yourself, and then hoping the person with whom you are angry will die. Oscar Wilde advised, "Always forgive your enemies; nothing annoys them so much." Be quick to forget unpleasant times and past injustices. Forgive yourself, as well.

- Look for opportunities to find quiet solace from the noisy and frenetic world. Silence renews the spirit, reduces tension, and naturally allows us to be mindful and in the moment.

Why Are the People of Denmark So Happy?

On a recent trip to Scandinavia, I spent about 48 hours in Copenhagen, Denmark. During my 2-day visit I traveled everywhere by bicycle as I had the pleasure of experiencing the unique charms of Copenhagen. The streets of this city are teeming with cyclists, and fully one-third of Danes commute to and from work each day by bike.

The evening I arrived there, my friends, Jorn and Bruce, met me downtown, where we enjoyed a memorable dinner. We were treated to a 10-course meal that included small servings of locally caught fish, grilled lamb, delicately prepared vegetables, and for dessert, fresh raspberries topped with a little cream. We drank hearty red wine with the meal and had decaf black coffee with dessert. By the time we finished it was almost 11:00 p.m., and it was time for Jorn to leave. So we walked him over to the central train station where he unlocked his slightly rusted very average-looking bike, and rolled it onto the train. About 15 minutes later this remarkable 75 year old gentleman rolled his bike off that train, and rode the 2 kilometers home, as he does every evening after work.

As it turns out, Denmark has, on average, the happiest people of any nation on the planet. They also have, next to Norway, the highest quality of life of any country, according to the Legatum Prosperity Index. Though I must say, you wouldn't know it to walk or cycle past them on the streets. They tend to be community minded, but are a stoic people by nature. When the scientists look below the surface to discover what makes Danes so contented despite living in a cloudy, windswept Scandinavian country, with its 17 hours of darkness during winter months, they come up with some interesting findings.

The Danes are happy and prosperous because they live and work with people they trust and so they feel safe and secure. They believe that they all are equal, and everyone's opinion is heard. On average, they work just 37 hours each week, and they pay about 70 percent of their earnings in taxes, but they seem to be okay with it. They take on average 6 weeks of vacation a year. Wealth and status are not revered in Denmark as they are in America. It appeared to me that few people were living lavish and wealthy lifestyles, but almost everybody seemed to be comfortable.

They enjoy the simple things in life, like the companionship of their family and friends, good food, and plenty of free time, enjoying outdoor activities like bicycling leisurely through the remarkably clean air and bustling, organized streets of Copenhagen. According to one Dane, "A rich person is not necessarily one with a lot of money, but rather the person who has a lot to be grateful for. The more people for which you develop a fondness, the richer your life will be."

They cultivate the art of living, and enjoy music, literature, food, and conversation and have cozy comfortable homes. They often belong to groups, clubs, associations, etc., and frequently volunteer. They tend to be fit and vigorous and enjoy being active out in nature. I came away from my short stay in Denmark thinking that we Americans could learn a thing or 2 from the Danes. Not that being happy is everything, but it does make life more meaningful, not to mention more fun.

Life Isn't About Waiting for the Storms to Pass; It's About Learning to Dance in the Rain

Steel, when tempered by fire, grows stronger. Bad weather makes good timber. Rough seas make tough and hardy sailors. During our lives, we all come through our own "fires" that can make us stronger, wiser, and more resilient. Joel Osteen says that we need to use the power of life's storms to take us to higher places. When everything seems to be coming against you, remember that airplanes take off into the wind. An eagle calmly rides fierce winds to soar above the tempest. Turbulent winds from storms in our lives can take us to new levels of our destiny, especially if we stay flexible, resilient, and optimistic in our thinking. I have countless patients who after discovering they had heart disease or even cardiovascular risk factors like diabetes or high blood pressure, responded to these threats by channeling their fear into motivation to eat right and exercise, and became stronger, more vigorous, and healthier than they had been in decades.

> "Most of the important things in the world have been ac-complished by people who have kept on trying when there seemed to be no hope at all."
> –Dale Carnegie

The Gift of Life: Donate Blood

Verner, an 82 year old with a severe, recurrent, life-threat-ening anemia told me before he died, "Over the past 5 months I have received 19 pints of blood from 19 different blood donors of varying races, ages, genders, sexual persuasions, and political views. The blood coursing through my vessels reminds me I am alive today because of the kindness of strangers, and that I have no right to be prejudiced towards anyone. We humans are really all one family, and we are all very dependent upon one another."

I have a relatively rare blood type, A-, and thus the local blood bank is often calling to remind me to donate when their sup-ply is running low. For the last 20 years, I have been donating a unit of blood 3 or 4 times a year. I like the idea that I might be helping someone in need, and I have always imagined that it somehow was good for me too—kind of like changing the oil in the car. In fact, some studies suggest that you can improve your long term cardiovascular health by giving blood regularly. Many of us, especially males and postmenopausal females, can gradually accumulate too much iron in the body. Too much iron stored in the body can wreak havoc throughout your system by generating free radical molecules that accelerate the aging process and increase the risks of cancer and heart disease.

Giving a unit of blood is an effective way to get rid of excess iron. It will lower your blood pressure, at least temporarily. Additionally, the screening process that you undergo each time you donate blood is a free mini-checkup that includes measurements of blood pressure, pulse, temperature, and blood tests to check for HIV, hepatitis, anemia, and high cholesterol. So rally your courage and roll up your sleeve. It's easier than you think, and the life you save might be your own.

9 Attitudes for Health and Contentment

In summary, let me suggest the following 9 attitudes and approaches to life that can improve your well-being, health, and contentment.

1. Work hard and be nice; and play hard too. We have found that if we don't make time to play, we have a more difficult time working hard and being nice on a consistent day-to-day basis.

2. Take what life throws at you and do your best—it's really all we can do. Everyone has issues. Figure out what your problem areas are and address them. It's never too late to make a change for the better. Turn your weaknesses into strengths by focusing on improving them.

3. There are no short cuts in life. Health, happiness, and success do not happen by accident. The more you do to take good care of yourself today, the luckier you will be in regards to your health, and the brighter your future will be. And the simple un-avoidable truth is that as the decades accumulate past age 30, the harder a person has to work at staying optimally healthy and youthful. But the dividends yielded from the investments of your time, energy, and expense are impressive and invaluable: you can stay youthful, vibrant, and fully alive to a much older age than ever before possible.

4. Try not to feel sorry for yourself or dwell on what you don't have. Self-pity is a waste of time and energy, and will take you no-where but down. It is up to you to create your own happiness.

5. Knowledge is power, especially with respect to your health and well-being. Be vigilant and proactive about your health issues.

6. Nothing rejuvenates your mind and body like exuberant play. Make it a priority to do something physical that feels like fun every day.

7. Never consider yourself too old to do things you enjoyed in your younger years. When you resign yourself to this defeatist attitude, it becomes a self-fulfilling prophecy. You are only as old as you think you are. Think younger and you will look, feel and act younger.

> "The great man is he who has not lost
> his child-heart."
> -Confucius

8. Laugh and smile more. Try to spend more time with optimistic, kind, grateful, and contented people and anyone who makes you happy. Avoid hanging around depressed, rude, resentful,

pessimistic, and mean-spirited people. Attitudes and behaviors are contagious—get exposed to upbeat individuals so you can catch their enthusiasm, and try to avoid being over-exposed to people with toxic outlooks on life.

9. Financial worry is consistently reported to be a major source of emotional stress for many people. Those who report high levels of money-related stress have been found to be at increased risk for a wide array of serious illnesses such as heart attacks, high blood pressure, ulcers, migraines, back pain, anxiety, and depression. The cost of excess debt and financial worries is not just the exorbitant interest payments you make to Visa and the bank. The true cost can be the toll that debt-related angst takes on the quality of your life and relationships, and even your health. Studies indicate that the amount of money you owe does not predict depression and health problems as well as how much you worry about it. So if debt is a major source of worry for you, take a cue from the frugal generation that survived the Great Depression. Make it a priority to keep your debt at a level that does not keep you awake tossing and turning at night.

CHAPTER 23

Healthy Pleasures: Feel Good without the Guilt

Mark Twain was dead wrong when he quipped, "The only way to keep your health is to eat what you don't want, drink what you don't like, and do what you'd rather not." Turns out that staying healthy isn't all about deprivation; many of life's most exquisite pleasures are among the best things for your well-being and longevity. So you can stop feeling guilty about these habits—they will make your life not just more pleasant, but also longer and healthier.

Play Like Your Life Depends on It

We don't stop playing because we get old; we get old because we stop playing. Physical activity is super good for you; problem is, we tend to think of exercise as an unpleasant chore—a workout doesn't connote fun. On the other hand, the more you can move your body with joy, or enthusiasm, or passion, the healthier, happier, and more youthful you will be. So make it a point to inject some physical play into each day.

Hands down, your best choice for combining exercise and pleasure is sexual activity. Having sexual relations with your spouse or significant other releases powerful feel-good hormones like oxytocin and endorphins. These not only make you happy, but they also strengthen psychological bonds and promote intimacy. Feeling emotionally connected on an intimate level to another person provides powerful benefits to your mental and physical health.

Even just a kiss can make us feel more connected; a deep and soulful kiss is like saying, "I love you" without words. The experts say that even if you have been together a long time, kissing each other like you mean it, is important. Marilyn Anderson, author of *Never Kiss a Frog*, says, "Put your whole body into the kiss. Without words, your lips should say, 'Baby, there's more where that came from!'" Getting frisky on a regular basis has been shown to improve immunity and is linked to better cardiovascular health. Of course sexual activity in the wrong settings can cause all sorts of serious health problems and social predicaments, so it is important to practice safe sex.

Dancing is another great option to move just for the fun of it. Dance classes, dancing with your partner, or even dancing alone with your iPod—or whenever the spirit moves you (like I catch myself doing more these days)—are fun and easy ways to get fit and happy without even trying.

When you were a kid you probably loved to play active games, often outside, not because it was good for you, but because fun is, well...fun. So find sports you can do with your friends and make it a priority to play as often as possible. Playing outdoors, even just walking with friends, is especially great for your health and well-being.

Vacation: A Luxury You Can't Afford to Do Without

Chronic stress is much more than just emotional strain; accumulating evidence indicates that it's harmful to nearly all of your organs, especially your heart and brain. An alarming 75 percent of all doctor visits are at least in part triggered by stress.

High blood pressure, irregular heartbeats, heart attacks, headaches, gastrointestinal problems, sleep disorders, gum disease, and even sudden cardiac arrest are among the countless health problems that are linked to emotional stress. Even obesity has been shown to occur more often in employees who report being stressed at work than in those who do not feel job-related strain. Cortisol, a stress hormone, may be one of the culprits; it stimulates cravings for high-carb junk food and predisposes to increased deposits of belly fat. Too much stress also tends to make us lethargic and depressed, and thus more likely to spend our free time sprawled out on a couch staring mindlessly at a television, for instance.

Although regular vacations may seem like an unnecessary extravagance, the scientific evidence suggests that they not only make us happier, but also reduce risks for illness, and may even improve life expectancy. One study of 12,000 men at high risk for heart disease, found that compared to those who didn't vacation regularly, those who took vacations at least once yearly were 32 percent less likely to die from all causes, and 39 percent less likely to die from cardiovascular disease. Vacays, as my kids call them, are great for rejuvenating us and recharging our enthusiasm. Especially during stressful times it is important to take a break from work and get away with loved ones or friends to a relaxing and fun spot. Personally, I find that even just making plans for a vacation, and anticipating a fun and adventurous trip, makes me feel enthused and happy. Ideally you should take several vacations throughout the year so you always have something to be looking forward to.

Sure, kick back and get plenty of rest, but also include a lot of hearty exercise in your vacations plans. Physical activity stimulates brain chemicals that make us happy, energized and relaxed. Fit is the new fun, and daily exercise is a sure-fire strategy to make you feel more attractive, self-confident, joyful, smarter and more stress-proof.

If you live in a region where winter is a cold and snowy season, make it a point to get away to a warm and sunny climate for at least 1 week sometime during the December through March timeframe. It's important for boosting vitamin D levels as well as your sense of well-being.

Sleep: Get Your ZZZZZs

No controversy here—sleep might feel like an indulgent luxury, but 7½ to 9 hours deep restorative sleep on a nightly basis is one of the most important habits you can cultivate to ensure a long and vigorous life. Sleep costs nothing, has zero drawbacks, and besides feeling wonderfully rejuvenating, also boosts your energy, improves your memory and creativity, strengthens the immune system, improves your mood, and helps you to stay lean and fit.

On the other hand, sleep deprivation causes high blood pressure, high glucose and excess belly fat, not to mention a cranky and irritable disposition. A recent study of 500,000 people showed that those who routinely slept less than 6 hours nightly had a substantially increased risk for heart attack, stroke and diabetes. By the way, it's normal to sleep for 3 or 4 hours deeply for the first half of the night, and then awaken for a period of time before you fall back to sleep for the second half of your night's slumber. Don't fret over this interlude; just lie quietly in your comfortable bed and let your mind wander. And rather than counting sheep, count your blessings.

If you're having trouble sleeping, rather than resorting to prescription medications, which can be habit-forming and cause fatigue the next day, try taking aspirin, 81 mg, and/or sustained-release melatonin, 3 mg, about 15 to 30 minutes before bedtime. These are safe, effective, and non-habit forming over-the-counter sleep aids. Napping is another treat that turns out to be good for your heart and your attitude, so don't feel guilty about a little mid-day snooze.

Chocolate as Health Food?

Paul is a real estate broker who was very distraught about the plummeting values of his properties during the early months of the great recession in 2008. In his stressed mental state he downed almost a whole 1-lb bag of M&Ms®, and a few hours later drove himself to our emergency room in the throes of a heart attack. He consumed over 2,000 calories of sugar and saturated fats that spiked his sugar and triglycerides, causing a sudden worsening of the silent but deadly inflammation that had been festering in his coronary arteries, which in turn triggered a sudden blood clot that blocked flow entirely into his RCA (right coronary artery). Fortunately Paul managed to drive himself to our hospital just in time; within a few seconds of stumbling through the doors of the Emergency Department while clutching his chest, his heart stopped and he collapsed unconscious to the floor. The nurses and doctors pounced on him immediately and shocked him out of ventricular fibrillation—a lethal cardiac rhythm. He was then taken urgently to the cardiac catheterization lab where a stent was placed to open his RCA blockage. Today, Paul is healthier, happier, and more fit than he has been in decades. Did I mention that he lost his taste for M&Ms® after his near-death-by-chocolate experience?

Paul's story aside, chocolate isn't pure evil. Dark chocolate, in small quantities, may benefit the health of the blood vessels by making the arteries more relaxed and responsive. Studies generally indicate that the antioxidants in dark chocolate lower blood pressure. But don't use these findings to go out and binge on chocolate cake or any of the countless choices of high-calorie chocolate flavored junk foods. Steve, one of our patients who struggles with his weight told me during an office visit, "I read that dark chocolate is recommended as a healthy food, so I have been eating about a bowl of Ben & Jerry's chocolate ice cream every night. I'm disappointed that my weight, blood pressure, and cholesterol have just gotten worse." I'm pretty sure I don't need to explain why chocolate ice cream is not going to provide the antioxidant benefits of dark chocolate. Do I?

Many of the studies on chocolate are sponsored by the candy companies and may turn out to be junk science. Make no mistake, too much chocolate will make you fat, not healthy, and some studies link chocolate to osteoporosis (weak bones). Our bottom line on chocolate: okay to enjoy as a treat if you are not in the weight-loss mode, but not more than about once or twice a week, and even then, only high quality dark chocolate that is 70 percent or higher in cacao, and only in very small quantities—about 10 to 12 grams, which is approximately the equivalent of 2 Hershey's Kisses (Hershey's does make a 70 percent chocolate called Bliss Dark Chocolate) . These are the doses and kinds of chocolate that have been found to be potentially beneficial to the arteries.

Socializing with Friends and Family

Over the past decade a whole new field of science has emerged focusing on the benefits of strong social ties and a positive attitude. Friendships are good for your health, especially if you spend time with well-adjusted, generally happy people who have your best interests in mind. Indeed, attitudes are communicable, for the better and for the worse, so try to gravitate to people who have a positive outlook on life.

An important study confirmed that having a sunny outlook and seeing the glass as half-full may help you live a longer and healthier life. This study, published in February 2011 in the *Archives of Internal Medicine*, evaluated the psychological and physical health of nearly 3,000 heart patients and found that those with an optimistic outlook were about 30 percent more likely to be alive after 15 years than their pessimistic counterparts. In essence, optimism is as powerful as the best drugs we have for improving the long-term health and survival of cardiac patients. So try to look at the bright side.

Speaking of attitudes that promote well-being and longevity, gratitude bestows powerful benefits to our mental and physical health. Individuals who feel grateful report more energy and optimism, better relationships, and happier moods, with lower risks for alcoholism and depression. A grateful heart is linked with higher wages, better sleep and fitness, and stronger immunity. I spoke with a friend whose wife is dying of cancer, and as distraught as he was, he said, "Sometimes when I am alone, I just want to scream and cry about how unfair this is, but then I remind myself just to be grateful that such a warm and loving person came into in my life, even if it wasn't for long enough time." I was inspired by his courage and strength and it reminded me to not take all my blessings for granted.

Enjoy Some High-Fat Foods

Although various experts have been scolding us for decades about eating fatty foods, they were wrong. Even today it is common to hear advice to follow a low-fat diet. The truth is that some high-fat foods are among the healthiest things you can eat. Plus full-fat foods taste better, and help to keep you full longer. Avocados, extra virgin olive oil, naturally oily fish like salmon and sea bass, and nuts are all high in fat—the healthy kinds. Unlike the nasty saturated fats present in greasy hamburger and other fatty meats, as well as in high-fat dairy, the good fats will lower risk of heart attack and stroke, and are good for your brain and joints. Some diets, including the Flat Belly Diet, focus on eating a modest amount of foods containing healthy fat with each meal. You should try to eat about 30 percent of your daily calories from healthy fats.

Massage Therapy

Getting a rubdown not only feels good, it also reduces stress and lowers blood pressure. People who are touched regularly, especially in a gentle and affectionate manner, tend to be healthier and happier. Human touch can confer powerful healing and soothing effects on a person, particularly when they are feeling stressed. If you don't have the time or the money to spend at the spa, consider getting in the habit of using healing touch therapy with your significant other. Studies show that women, after being massaged at least 2 times weekly by their partners, reported feeling less depression, anxiety, and anger; not surprisingly, their partners reported better moods too.

Your Morning Buzz: Coffee and Tea

No morning regrets—coffee and tea (hold the cream and sugar) are among the healthiest beverages you can drink. Both coffee and tea are loaded with disease-fighting, anti-aging antioxidants and they are essentially calorie free. Drinking 4 cups of coffee per day reduces risk of diabetes and neuro-degenerative diseases including Parkinson's and Alzheimer's. Black coffee and green tea are turning out to be an amazingly beneficial drinks for preventing everything from high blood pressure, high cholesterol and diabetes, to reducing risks for brain diseases and some cancers. They rev up your metabolism and help you to exercise harder and longer. Be careful about getting too much caffeine, and avoid caffeinated versions of coffee or tea after about mid-afternoon.

Sun Bathing

As a kid growing up near the Canadian border, I remember feeling a euphoric natural high when the warming rays of sun would make their reappearance in mid-March. At the end of a long, cold, and dark winter I would go out in my shorts and T-shirt, even when the temperatures were still in the 40s, look up at the sun, close my eyes and bask in the wonderful goodness of those golden rays. It was like scratching an intense itch. In fact this need for the sun is a powerful instinct that compels us to soak up the sunlight when it's available to ensure that we get our vitamin D levels back into the normal healthy ranges. Sunlight in the non-winter months will stimulate your skin to produce large amounts of vitamin D, which is perhaps the most important vitamin of all. Keeping your vitamin D levels up may help to prevent cancers, osteoporosis, heart disease, infections, depression, and diabetes, to name just a few of its many health benefits. Be careful to avoid sunburn; too much sun can cause premature skin aging and skin cancers. Limit your unprotected, midday, non-winter sun exposure to 15 to 20 minutes daily, after which you should put on sunscreen.

A Glass of Wine with Dinner

Raise a glass to toast the health benefits of your nightly wine habit, as long as you keep it to 1 if you are a woman and up to 2 per day for a man. As we've discussed, alcohol in small daily quantities reduces heart disease and diabetes as well as exercise or the best of our medications. The devil is in the dosing—at quantities greater than 2 drinks per day, the risks for a host of adverse health effects rise in proportion to the amount of alcohol consumed.

CHAPTER 24

Sex:
Not Just for Making Babies Anymore

"Love doesn't make the world go round.
Love is what makes the ride worthwhile."
–Franklin Jones

Brad, one of my patients, confided to me during an office visit, "I've been divorced for 3 years, but I still had been seeing my ex-wife once a week. Recently she told me she is seeing someone else, and doesn't want to be going out on dates with me anymore. Strangely, this has somehow this made me feel better; like I have some closure and I can finally move on with my life. My mood is so much better, like a weight has been lifted off my chest." I told him, "That's great Brad. Now maybe you can go out and find a new someone special for yourself; to make your heart happy again." As his eyes welled up with tears, Brad asked, "Is my heart strong enough for that now?" I replied, "To be honest, those are not the kind of heart problems that I am trained to diagnose or treat, but my intuition tells me that yes, Brad you have a very good heart in more ways than one, and love might be exactly what you need more than anything else right now."

Sure, you have always known that sex can put a twinkle in your eye and a spring in your step, but the latest science shows that an active sex life can also confer a multitude of impressive benefits to health, well-being, and longevity for both men and women (assuming that safe sex practices are followed so as to minimize the risk of contracting sexually transmitted infections). Men and women who report having sexual activity at least once or twice a week have improved life expectancy, lower risks for heart attack and stroke, improved immune system function and lower risk of prostate cancer.

If nothing else, sex is an entertaining and pleasurable form of exercise . . . a vigorous 30-minute romp will burn up to 200 calories—about the same as walking 2 miles, or running 15 minutes on a treadmill. It also is a workout for the muscles of the pelvis, thighs, buttocks, arms, neck and chest. Sexual activity and orgasm boost production of testosterone estrogen and oxytocin, which help to build stronger bones and muscles and improve emotional well-being. Sexual intercourse stimulates the production of prolactin, which has been linked to improvements in mood, psychological bonding, and even your sense of smell.

So make it a priority to invest the time and energy into maintaining an active sex life with the person you love. As he was getting older, when asked about his sex life Jack LaLanne, the 'Godfather of fitness' joked, "My wife and I still make love almost every night: almost on Monday, almost on Tuesday, almost on Wednesday..." Sex is exercise that feels more like playtime than a workout; and it offers unique and impressive benefits for your heart, brain, attitude, and even longevity.

Are Viagra, Levitra, or Cialis Safe for Your Heart?

This is one of the more common questions I get from my male patients. Or sometimes it's the significant other who is worried that one of these drugs for erectile dysfunction (ED) might stress their partner's heart. In fact, for most people these ED drugs are very safe and highly effective.

Sex is designed by nature to be one of life's most exquisite pleasures. Physical intimacy bonds us to our partner like nothing else, and helps to cement and maintain a close, personal, and loving connection. Having an intimate long-term relationship is one of the most important predictors of someone who will stay healthy and happy despite the stresses and strains that life inevitably throws at us along our journey. So by helping to improve sexual ability in men, these ED drugs can be helpful to their heart health and overall well-being.

> "An older gentleman was out fishing when he heard a small voice say, 'Pick me up.' He looked down and saw a frog on the riverbank. The frog said, 'Kiss me, and I'll turn into a beautiful princess.' The man thought for a moment, then reached over and carefully placed the frog in his pocket. The frog exclaimed, 'What are you doing, don't you want a gorgeous young wife?' The man answered, 'Frankly, at this point in my life,
> I'd really rather have a talking frog.'"
> -Anonymous

A Curious Side Effect

These drugs were discovered by accident about 20 years ago when scientists were looking for a drug to treat heart disease. This particular drug (eventually named Viagra) turned out to dilate blood vessels particularly well in the penis. As they say, the rest is history, and this drug alone has grown into a billion-dollar-per-year blockbuster.

The take-home message is that these drugs dilate blood vessels which in general is good for your heart. Check in with your physician before starting one of the drugs just to be sure. And be careful not to use nitroglycerin-type medicines in combination with Viagra, Levitra, or Cialis, because they might lower your blood pressure too much.

These erectile dysfunction medicines are relatively expensive, at about $15 to 20 per pill. But as the wife of one of my patients put it, "It's about the same as what we would pay to go see a movie, and sex is much more fun and way better for improving my mood."

New Thinking on Hormone Replacement Therapy

Estrogen for Post-Menopausal Women?

I asked one of my patients, "Darlene, have you gone through menopause yet?" She replied, "No, but I'm feel like I'm down to my last half-dozen eggs, and I'm sure they are scrambled by now."

Stephanie is a 51-year-old woman who recently came to see me complaining that her heart was skipping and racing. Although these spells would only last for a few seconds, she found them distracting and worrisome. She also had been waking up in the middle of the night with drenching sweats and a flushed feeling in her face.

Stephanie confided that she was feeling generally more irritable and just less happy than usual in recent months. When we checked her labs, we found that her bad cholesterol was 20 points higher and her good cholesterol was 5 points lower than was normal for her. As we both suspected, her hormone levels showed that she was in menopause. After about 40 years of cyclic estrogen production, her ovaries were calling it quits.

We've Come a Long Way, Baby!

A decade ago most doctors would not have thought twice before starting Stephanie on hormone replacement therapy with estrogen and progesterone. The cover of *TIME* magazine in the mid

'90s proclaimed post-menopausal hormone therapy as the fountain of youth for women.

This field was thrown into turmoil when a large and scientifically valid study called the Women's Health Initiative (WHI) published its results in 2002 showing that estrogen, especially when used with progesterone, increased the risk of blood clots, heart attacks, and strokes. The previously popular strategy of estrogen for menopausal women took a sudden U-turn, and this practice has been decidedly out of fashion among physicians and patients for the past decade. Yet, reassuring new findings and innovative options are changing our thinking about this complex and important issue of estrogen replacement for women past menopause.

What's New in Hormone Replacement

The latest data out from the WHI and other studies suggests that hormones for the first 10 years after menopause are not only safe, but also may reduce the risk of death from any cause. A recently reported study of over 700,000 women found that topical (the medical term for treatment applied to the skin) estrogen therapy is safer for a woman's heart than the pill form of estrogen.

Hormone pills that you swallow have to pass through the liver where the estrogen is metabolized into compounds that are different from the estrogens that are produced in the ovaries. On the other hand, topical estrogen is absorbed through the skin straight into the bloodstream, similar to the natural release of hormones from the ovaries directly into the circulation.

Patches for the skin can deliver estrogen at doses that are safe, effective, and easy. The most popular patches are designed to be applied to the skin of the torso, arm, or thigh, and changed every 3 to 7 days. If you are considering hormone therapy for post-menopausal issues, remember: safety may be skin deep.

Bio-identical Hormones

Bio-identical hormone therapy is another hot topic in this field. Many of the old studies, including the WHI trial, used oral hormone pills which often contain a variety of different estrogens. Some of these are not normally made by human females. It is much more logical to use the precise form of estrogen (17-beta estradiol) that your ovaries made before you went through menopause. Today, it is easy to find estrogen compounds that are exactly the same, biochemically, as the hormones produced by a healthy young woman's ovaries.

Dr. Marie Griffin is a friend and endocrinologist who is very bright and knowledgeable on the topic of hormone therapy for women. Dr. Griffin says, "With a life expectancy of nearly 90 years for American women today, they are spending about 40 years with deficient or absent sex hormones. Are their brains, bones, GI tracts, muscles, uro-genital tracts, etc., ready for that? Often our male counterparts' testosterone levels fall gradually through the decades to low-normal levels, but not to zero! And when they come in with low testosterone, do we tell them to tough it out because they might get prostate cancer or could have a drop in their HDL (cardio-protective) cholesterol? Heck no! We put most of them on testosterone because it's so central to their health and well-being. I think there's an unintentional double standard in this issue. Estrogen should be offered to post-menopausal women after having a balanced discussion about the risks versus benefits of estrogen therapy."

Weighing the Risks Versus Benefits of Estrogen Replacement

Many women feel better emotionally and physically when they use hormones early after menopause. Improvements in mood, energy, skin youthfulness, memory, cholesterol levels, sex drive, and bone health are all potential benefits of post-menopausal estrogen. No wonder so many women are interested in hormone replacement! However, there are downsides to consider. Estrogen can increase the risks of breast cancer, blood clots, heart attacks, and strokes, especially with high-dose hormonal therapy used for over 10 years.

My friend and collaborator Dr. David Bell, an endocrinologist from Alabama who is a leading expert on issues related to hormones and heart disease says, "Estrogen therapy around the time of menopause and for up to 10 years afterwards appears to prevent heart disease. In contrast, estrogen in older women (those over 65), especially those with established cardiovascular disease, can increase the risk of heart attack and stroke."

The issues surrounding hormone therapy for women are complex and need to be considered on a case-by-case basis. So, if you have questions about this, talk it over with your doctor, though probably not your cardiologist, since we generally neither prescribe nor follow women's hormone replacement therapy issues closely.

Incidentally, Stephanie's gynecologist did start her on a low-dose estrogen patch and her palpitations and other menopausal symptoms improved markedly.

Is Estrogen Replacement Right for You?

Here are a few points to discuss with your doctor if you are currently using, or are considering starting, post-menopausal estrogen replacement therapy:

1. Use the lowest dose possible.

2. Try to use topical (applied to skin) or intra-vaginal hormones.

3. Ask about bio-identical (human identical) estrogen therapy.

4. Estrogen replacement is safest for women in the first decade after menopause starts; typically from age 50 to 60.

5. Avoid hormone therapy if you have a personal or family history of breast cancer, blood clots in the legs, stroke, or heart attack.

6. Have regular check-ups with your gynecologist, internist, endocrinologist, or family practice physician while on estrogen therapy.

CHAPTER 25

Secrets of Longevity

"Around here we don't look backward for very long. We
keep moving forward, opening new doors, and doing
new things, because we're curious…and curiosity keeps
leading us down new paths."
–Walt Disney

The Art of Aging Gracefully

Dorothy O'Keefe, my grandmother, lived to be 102. She was
a real inspiration for all who knew her. She was a big part of my life
especially when I lived with her for 4 years in her home in Grand
Forks, North Dakota, while attending college and medical school at
the University of North Dakota. She was such a kick; spunky, irrepressible, optimistic, with a great sense of humor and love of life.
Born in 1903, she came of age during the Roaring Twenties. She had
a strong faith, and always put family first. She never missed church
on Sunday morning, or having her 1 or 2 whiskeys every evening at
happy hour before dinner. Dorothy never looked back, had a self-
deprecating sense of humor and a toughness and resilience honed
during the Great Depression. One of her mottos was, "Tough times
don't last, but tough people do." During the decade of the 1930s she
was raising her 3 children while working full time and also caring for
her husband (my paternal grandfather) who was struggling to survive

tuberculosis and alcoholism. She was volunteering at her church and a local nursing home until age 90. At her 102nd birthday party, our then 5 year old, Caroline, asked, "Granny, what's the best thing about being 102?" Dorothy answered, "No peer pressure."

In 1950, only 3,000 people in the U.S. managed to hang in there to celebrate 100 birthdays; that number grew to 37,000 in 1990, according to the U.S. Census Bureau. By 2050, the number of 100-year-old Americans will grow to an astounding 1.1 million! Live right and you may someday see 100. Although many people think longevity is all about the genes, it's really only 25 percent due to heredity and 75 percent a function of your lifestyle, diet, attitude, and other factors largely under your control. To date, the longevity record (firmly documented) belongs to Jeanne Calment of Arles, France, a woman born in 1875. She passed away in 1997 at 122 years, 5 months, and 14 days. When asked what her secret was Jeanne replied, "Always keep your smile."

Every Body Dies, but Not Every Body Lives

A depressed 45-year-old man asked his doctor, "How long do you think I will live?" The doctor asked him, "Do you climb mountains, sky dive, or swim in the ocean?" The man answered, "No, I don't do anything risky." The doctor pressed him further. "Do you travel to exotic destinations?" "No, I never fly anywhere—too dangerous!" "Do you drink?" He responded, "No, I never touch the stuff." "Do you eat red meat or chocolate," the doctor asked? "Never," the man said. Finally the physician asked, "Do you enjoy sex?" "Not much anymore," he said. So, the doctor looked at him, shrugged and said, "Well then, honestly, I don't see why you should even care how long you have left to live."

We Americans are becoming healthier and healthier and are living longer and longer. Life expectancy has approximately doubled in the last century. And although experts have been predicting that the gains in longevity will plateau, the average lifespan keeps rising, and thanks to modern medicine, older people are healthier than ever.

Take Walter Breuning, a 112-year-old resident of Great Falls, Montana, for example. Walter recently took over the honor of being the oldest living person. He taught himself to read in the dim light of a flickering kerosene lantern, and cast his first presidential ballot for Woodrow Wilson. Every day Walter takes 1 baby aspirin and eats only 2 meals. He still enjoys walking and he is most grateful for his health. "If you're in good health, you've got everything," he says. Longevity did not run in Breuning's family, at least until Walter came along. Both of his parents were dead by age 50, and his 4 siblings died in their 70s. Breuning's secrets to longevity included staying active in body and mind, practicing moderation and treating others with kindness and respect.

My grandmother Alice used to say, "It's a great life if you don't weaken." She lived on the second floor of an apartment building without an elevator, never owned a car, walked everywhere, and even carried her groceries home from the neighborhood market in her little hometown of Crookston, Minnesota. Indeed, Alice was a strong woman emotionally and physically, and she often said that she had 85 good years. The end of her high-quality life came shortly after she decided she could no longer climb up and down the long, steep staircase to her apartment. Shortly thereafter, Alice moved into a retirement facility where she learned that when she quit doing the hard things, the easy things in her life became hard. She settled into a wheelchair, where she spent most of the last 8 years of her life.

Today, the fastest growing segment of the population is over age 85. Studies indicate that, contrary to popular belief, most people tend to get happier as the years go by beyond middle age. Satisfaction and happiness usually are very high for people in their 20s, and then we tend to become less happy until about age 45, when we start to get happier again; within about a decade most people are as happy or happier than they were in their 20s. The 2 main threats to your continued happiness and well-being during the second half of your life are social isolation and the loss of your good health. But beware, both of these threats are very real and so you need to be proactive about avoiding them. For example, although the age-adjusted death rate from cardiovascular disease has fallen by two-thirds over the past 25 years, if you are a man age 50 or older without a history of heart trouble, you still have about a 50 percent chance of developing heart disease during your lifetime, and the risk for a woman is about 40 percent. Also at age 50 your chance of developing diabetes during the duration of your lifetime is 33 percent for men and 40 percent for women.

Mary, a high-spirited 74-year-old widow, proclaimed, "I've decided that my goal is to die young... as late as possible." Like Mary, most of us are more concerned with the quality of our life rather than the sheer quantity of years we are alive. The latest research shows that being physically active from middle age on is the single best way not only to survive into old age, but also to thrive with vigor and joy. In November 2010 at the American Heart Association meeting, Dr. Jarett Berry presented data showing if you are physically active in mid-life, you double your chances of surviving to 85. Or stated in another way, if you are not fit in your 50s, your projected lifespan is almost a decade shorter than if you are fit in mid-life. More importantly, if you want to do more than just exist, daily exercise will preserve your physical vitality, mental sharpness, and overall quality of life more than anything else you can do. In this study of 1,765 men and women, being physically fit outperformed all other factors, even not smoking and having low blood pressure, as the best predictor of longevity.

Many Americans have fallen into the habit of taking the path of least effort, preferring to take a pill rather than getting up off the couch and get moving. This tendency to do less physical activity and become less fit each year after age 30 is a serious threat to overall health and happiness. National guidelines recommend 30 minutes or more a day of moderate activity, 5 days a week at least. Or if preferred, 20 minutes of high-intensity exercise 5 times a week. Also, try to include weight-training exercises for at least 20 minutes 2 times a week. Weight lifting lowers your post-workout and day-to-day blood pressures at least as well as cardio exercise.

Working Longer May Help You Live Longer

Recently I said to one of my patients, "It's been over 2 years since I last saw you. Hal, I know you are busy as an assistant funeral director, and I think it's great you are still working at age 75, but with your heart history, it's important that you be seen for an office visit at least once a year." Hal replied, "I suppose you're right. I know that I would much rather be seen than be viewed."

If you think retiring and saying goodbye forever to workday stress will improve your health, you're wrong. A recent study showed individuals who opted for full retirement experienced a 23 percent increase in difficulty performing daily activities, an 11 percent decline in mental health, and an 8 percent increase in illness, compared to those who continued to work at least part time.

Be a Work in Progress

Life is never static; it tends to be either in the growth mode or decay mode. You might think that you are a point in your life where you can afford to ease off and not work so hard at staying active mentally and physically. When we lose our drive, settle back, and aimlessly coast along, our physical and mental powers begin to atrophy. Work can motivate us to acquire new skills and knowledge, which helps ensure we will never stop growing. Okinawa is an island south of Japan that is home to perhaps the healthiest and longest lived people in the world. The Okinawans literally do not have word for retirement in their dialect. As people age they may change what they do, but they never completely retire.

Complacency is one of your worst enemies, and some stress in your life turns out to be a good thing. A job that requires you to use your body and your brain can keep you youthful. Studies show there are 4 essential components to staying healthy later in life: social connectedness, mental stimulation, physical activity, and a healthy diet. Continuing to work, even if it's part time or volunteer work, can help you make the first 3 happen.

I mentioned to my patient Jerry that he was in great shape for a 69 year old, and if he kept up his excellent diet and exercise, he could plan on at least another decade of a vigorous life, if not 2 or 3. He replied, "Really? In that case I am going to have to coax my wife out of retirement to make sure we don't run out of money."

No doubt, age takes a toll on some brain functions like reaction time, ability to multi-task, and short-term memory, but the latest research indicates that some brain functions actually improve with age. Living through decades of real life experiences instills a wisdom you can't find in a book and teaches us how to be more efficient in solving problems. You don't need to reinvent the wheel each time when you have seen it all before. In a profession like cardiology, this can be invaluable.

Dr. Barry Rutherford is one of my long time cardiology colleagues. Over 30 years ago, Dr. Rutherford, along with Dr. Geoffrey Hartzler, performed the first balloon angioplasty procedure to urgently open up an acutely blocked coronary artery, thereby restoring blood flow and oxygen to the heart, which dramatically reduces heart damage and often the saves the heart attack victim's life as well. He is an internationally recognized leader in the field of interventional cardiology, as he has been for decades, and today Barry remains on top of his game, physically and mentally. He exercises nearly every day, running 2 to 4 miles 3 days per week and lifting weights for 45 minutes nearly every day. He eats a very healthy diet and makes sure to get 8 hours of sleep nearly every night. Dr. Rutherford understands that with the demands of his job he needs to stay very fit and strong.

People today are living longer and more productive lives. Your community needs your talents, time, and wisdom as much as you need the emotional and financial perks from continued employment. I was speaking to an acquaintance who recently retired and I asked him, "Do you miss your work?" He replied, "Like a headache! I realized I was getting to know more and more about less and less. I decided I had better retire before I knew everything about nothing." He is now volunteering at a local grade school, taking classes at community college, spending hours exploring the internet, and planning upcoming trips.

> "The highest reward for a man's toil is not what he gets for it, but what he becomes by it."
> –John Ruskin

Bill is a primary care physician in a small town who is a friend of ours. He has an instinctive feel for the importance for continuing to work, something he has noticed in his own medical practice. At age 74, he continues to practice medicine 40 hours per week. He says that it challenges his mind and makes him enthused to get out of bed in the morning. On the other hand, Mary retired after 29 years as laboratory technician to become a guide and caretaker for a public garden/park. Now at age 62 she regularly leads guided walks through a state park pointing out the natural beauty of the native grasses, trees, and flowers.

Working longer is not always the path to better health, especially if your work is monotonous, stressful, and/or not intellectually stimulating or emotionally fulfilling. However, even if you retire from your primary occupation, find something to do that will present new challenges. Activities that offer you the chance to develop a sense of control and mastery are revitalizing for heart and soul, and can fortify your immune system.

When Your Life Has a Mission, Your Heart Is Happy

Harold is a very good friend who inspires us with his passion for life. He continues to work full time, though he retired from his paying job 15 years ago. Now he invests a great deal of his talent, energy, time, and money into an organization called Wayside Waifs.

> "Work like you don't need the money; love like you've never been hurt; dance like nobody's watching."
> –Satchel Paige

Harold is the chief executive officer of this not-for-profit animal shelter in Kansas City that is dedicated to finding loving and safe homes for untold numbers of stray or unwanted dogs and cats. Each morning Harold awakens knowing that his mission is making a difference for our community; bringing love, security, and companionship for thousands of animals each year, and perhaps even more benefits to the kind and generous people who adopt these pets. His eyes still sparkle with vitality and vigor, and he walks with a spring in his step. He thinks, acts, exercises, and lives like a man 30 years younger.

Harold will tell you that his love for family, friends, and Wayside Waifs is the driving force that fuels his passion for life. Six years ago he asked, "How's my health, Doc?" I replied, "Harold, if we are not someday celebrating your 100th birthday together, I will feel as though I have failed you." Now at age 93, Harold is as enthused and sharp as ever, and exercises every day; and we are already beginning to make plans for that centennial birthday bash I promised him.

Maybe we all can't contribute on the scale that Harold does, but even a little investment in the life around us has the power to bring strength and vitality to our lives. All living things are inter-connected through the great tree of life, and through our connec-tions with other life flows a vital force that sustains each of us just as the sap of a tree sustains its leaves. Whether or not we are aware of it, each one of us is woven into this network of life; and if we ignore this reality and become isolated and too self-centered, we grow ill and unhappy. Scientists studying this issue find that lonely, cut off, and depressed people tend to be unhealthy and die young-er. In other words, if you lose interest in life, life may lose interest in you. An isolated individual is a dead-end in the grand scheme of life. On the other hand, by contributing to and striving for the welfare of others, you can harness a mysterious and powerful en-ergy that ensures life will continue to thrive within you. Through its profound instinctive wisdom, life has a way of investing energy and vitality in those who are contributing positively to their community of life and withdrawing it from those who are not.

The islanders of Okinawa have an average lifespan of 86 years, making them one of the longest living and healthiest cul-tures in the world. Okinawans suffer 80 percent less heart disease, 75 percent less breast and prostate cancer, and 33 percent less dementia than their counterparts here in the U.S. The Okinawans attribute their exceptional longevity and vigor to a concept they call ikagai, or having a strong sense of purpose. They feel that an ongoing personal mission or destiny is essential for staying youth-ful and strong as they grow older.

Certainly, their traditional diet rich in vegetables and fish, and an active way of life, are factors in the Okinawans' excellent health. Yet, the people of this remarkable culture feel their longevity is most closely tied to ikagai, literally translated as "that which makes one's life worth living." A cause or a passion bigger than ourselves can help us transcend the selfish, introspective nature of an isolated human life, and can bring us lasting vitality and exceptional longevity. The Okinawans have a reciprocal support network of family, friends, and neighbors, and this brings a sense of belonging to these people. They tend to put family first and prioritize the cultivation and maintenance of lifelong friendships and social bonds.

"The answers to 3 questions will determine
your success or failure.
1. Can people trust you to do your best?
2. Are you committed to the task at hand?
3. Do you care about other people and show it?
If the answers to all these questions are yes,
there is no way you can fail."
–Lou Holtz

My mother, Leatrice, is a nurse by profession, and nurturing others has always come naturally for her. When my father passed away 10 years ago, she lost her best friend and soul mate. Understandably, she was depressed and anxious for a year or so afterwards, but she gradually regained her spark by re-investing her life in others. She volunteers regularly at both the nursing home and the church in our hometown of Grafton, North Dakota, a vibrant little community of 3,500 people near the Minnesota and Canadian borders. She regularly entertains company or travels to visit her family and friends, cares for a dog, and loves to garden (during the 5 months of the year that the temperature stays above freezing). Recently, she confided to us that she believes that she has been blessed with good health so that she can be there for many of her friends and neighbors who are getting older and sometimes find themselves struggling with serious health issues. Leatrice has a gentle, happy, and compassionate manner, and she spends her days providing good humor, hope, and kindhearted support for her friends and family, and in this way she finds strength and peace of mind for herself. To me, she has always seemed like the closest thing I have ever known to an angel, though I suppose it's natural for a person to feel that way about his or her own mother.

Here's the critical factor: no outside entity determines whether or not you are still important to the web of life, you do. It's your own being, conscious or subconscious, that judges whether you are still a dynamic life force that needs to continue to prosper. Living with a sense of purpose sends a signal to your brain that says, "I still matter," and this engenders attitudes and actions that resonate throughout your being, revitalizing your body, reinvigorating your mind, realigning your hormones, and helping you to thrive.

"Don't undermine your worth by comparing yourself with others. It is because we are different that each of us is special."
–Nancye Sims

Want to grow stronger? Give your energy to someone or some cause beyond yourself. Want to be happier? Stop worrying so much about your own self-interests and try to make someone else's life happier or easier. You don't have to change the world; you just need have lunch with a friend, or volunteer to help out with a cause that inspires you.

Joan's father Leonard, who lived to be 94 years old, used to say, "Keep on walkin' and keep on squawkin'; and don't look back." Indeed, a recent study found that people who made a habit of visiting with acquaintances, either in person or by phone, were significantly protected from Alzheimer's disease. Take good care of the people you love; happiness doesn't come from possessions or power, but instead from the relationships you develop with the people in your life whom you love and respect.

Tend a garden, or walk your dog, or feed the birds, or give your elderly neighbor a ride to the grocery store. You get what you give—it's one of the fundamental laws of nature, and it is a force that animates life. Tap into it and you will thrive and prosper; ignore it and you may wither like the leaf that becomes disconnected from its tree.

Brighten Your Future and Safeguard Your Well-Being

Chill out, man. Stress can wreak havoc on your system, from your brain and heart to your digestive tract and sexual function. Being alive means dealing with stress, so we all need to discover and cultivate healthy coping strategies that will work for us. My bright and beautiful sister Katie is one of my favorite people on Earth. She was dragged down in her 20s by a cocaine and prescription narcotics habit that devastated her emotional and physical health, and came within a few heart beats of losing her life at a young age. With the help of family and support groups she beat her addiction and rebuilt her spirituality, emotional resilience, and self-esteem.

Over the decade since then, Katie has completed her Master's degree in counseling, and has been helping others conquer their chemical demons. In the process she has become healthier and happier than ever; instead of relying upon cigarettes or other chemicals for stress relief, she exercises vigorously almost every day, and focuses on cultivating her spirituality. She runs with her dog, or lifts weights, or does yoga or Pilates with her friends; and like the rest of her siblings, she loves to hike in the Colorado mountains. For both Katie and me, there is nothing like vigorous climbing through the thin air, spectacular scenery, and blue skies to leave you feeling as though God is smiling down upon you.

Our personal relationships and our health are our 2 most valuable assets in life. Without these 2 essentials, we have nothing. When you feel battered by storms in your life, shipwrecked, left for dead, drifting aimlessly in a vast ocean of problems, connect with the people around you like your very survival depends upon it. Because it is not an exaggeration to state that the network of personal connections you cultivate with your friends, family, co-workers and community will be the life raft that will keep you alive, safe and sound, during the tough times. Those relationships will also keep you happy and healthy throughout your life. Women by nature are usually more adept than men at nurturing their personal relationships, which is one of the reasons they tend to outlive their male counterparts. Make it a priority to build a network of support by taking time to enjoy and appreciate the people in your life. And remember if you want to have a friend, you have to be a friend. Call, text, or e-mail your parents, children and friends often. Go out of your way to be kind, considerate, and interested in others around you, and consciously work at building and maintaining relationships: nothing will be more important for your happiness or health and well-being in the long run.

Invest your time, energy, and disposable income into experiences more than material things. A new car might make you happy for a short time, but it's a fleeting happiness. If you really want to increase the joy and meaning in your life, try to think of your time here on Earth as a great adventure to be shared and enjoyed with your companions. Experiences you share with your friends and family will add much more happiness and value to your life than material things you purchase. Learn to say no and only do things that bring you joy and wonder. Warren Buffet, widely considered to be one of the best investors in modern time, said in response to a question regarding his formula for success, "Say no to almost everything." If you don't prefer to do it or if it's likely to add undue stress to your life, learn to say no. You cannot do it all, nor can you please everyone. Set your priorities, and make sure one of them is setting aside plenty of time to invest in your own health and happiness.

Discover healthy (and legal, preferably) ways to inject some euphoria into your life—and then make it a part of your daily routine. Make a point of doing something kind and considerate for your family and friends or even a stranger. Tend a garden and care for the plants in your yard. Growing plants will revitalize your own health and well-being, even if they never make it to your dinner table. Take the long view. If something that is bothering you today won't matter 5 years from now—don't lose sleep over it. Don't take your life so seriously—it's not permanent. Strive to be curious and open-minded; never stop exploring and discovering. If you don't already know, learn how to use a computer. The internet is a universe, or rather a cyberspace, full of useful and fun information about whatever it is that fascinates you.

Fuel your body with the good stuff and avoid excess and toxic habits. One of the surest ways to make animals and humans live longer and healthier lives is to reduce calorie intake to match their energy expenditure. It is especially true if you also increase your consumption of anti-aging and disease-fighting nutrients by eating more fresh, unprocessed, whole foods like those found in nature. Don't eat unless you feel definite hunger. It is the mindless downing of massive amounts of junk food calories that causes most people to get fat. Shake your salt habit. As a society, we consume far too much salt. If everyone cut their intake to one-half that, or about 2,000 mg per day, it would save 150,000 lives each year! We would have to put every adult in America on a statin cholesterol drug, or get most of the smokers to quit permanently, to make this big of an impact on heart attacks, strokes, and deaths. The best way to avoid sodium is to eat more fruits, vegetables, nuts, berries, and to avoid processed foods and cook at home. Skip soups, deli meats, chips, bread, and crackers, too! Don't smoke. If you do smoke, quit as often as you need to. Electronic cigarettes are also an extremely effective and surprisingly safe way of stopping smoking.

Time, Not Money, Is the True Currency of Life

How do you want to spend the minutes, hours, days, years, and decades of your life? We want you to do anything and everything that your heart desires. Sadly, for many people, suboptimal health limits their options, as well as the quality and quantity of their years. Take a look around you; how many of your friends and family are overweight or obese, tired or depressed, shuffling listlessly from the bed to the chair to the doctor's office and back home? This is not how you were meant to live. Do you remember how you felt when you were 10 years old? Nothing ever made you stop and think, "I wish I could still do that." You were brimming with energy and enthusiasm for life. Or as an open-minded, curious, playful, physically sturdy, and emotionally resilient 21 year old, when you would jump at the chance to travel to a new destination without a second thought, or maybe stay up late dancing with a life of the party attitude. Your hormones were in their ideal ranges, which meant you had a high sex drive, strong muscles and bones, a flat belly, and a sharp mind. You slept deeply and awakened fully refreshed and recharged.

It is possible to regain the vim and vigor of your youth—you can be youthful in body and spirit far beyond your years, more so than any prior generation in the 150 thousand years that humans have walked the Earth. We have the knowledge and technology—

you just need to make it a priority to heed the advice in these pages. It will involve taking the best of both worlds.

We believe that time is the most valuable commodity in our lives. Time, not money, is the true currency of life. Each of us gets only so many hours and days; and we try to remind ourselves and our children that time is precious and not to be wasted. We suspect none of us will be on our death beds expressing regrets like, "If only I had watched more reality TV." Being alive is about experiencing your own real life and making a positive difference in your circle of influence, whether it's socializing with or helping your family and friends, being active and learning new things, meeting new people, or exploring new places.

Yet, it is hard to be fully engaged in life when you aren't feeling your best. This is why taking care of yourself is so critically important. If you overeat the wrong kinds of foods, you will pay for it during the next several hours as your system bogs down under an immediate flood of free radicals, stress chemicals, and hormones, impairing the performance of both brain and body, which can ruin the rest of your day. Additionally, a sedentary lifestyle is a downward spiral—the less you do, the less you feel like doing, and before long, the less you are capable of doing. Similarly, when you are sleep deprived, life can feel less enjoyable, and problems can seem more overwhelming. Fortunately, you can bring this vicious cycle to a screeching halt and turn it into a virtuous cycle that builds health and vigor.

Increasingly, it is becoming apparent that if we are interested in improving our health span (the quantity of years of life lived in good health) we cannot rely on any one magic bullet, whether it be a single supplement, a specific food, special juice, or solitary lifestyle change. Instead our health span can be extended through the adoption of a number of key steps, including regular physical exercise, adequate sleep, stress reduction, sensible sun exposure, vitamin D and omega 3 supplementation, avoidance of excess alcohol use, and staying away from tobacco altogether. Additionally, to maximize your health span, it is essential that you adopt a diet like the one followed by our hunter–gatherer ancestors. We have been genetically designed by natural selection to thrive upon a diet of fresh fruits and vegetables, nuts and seeds, fish, shellfish, eggs, lean fresh meat, and water. In fact, scientific studies show this diet is superior to virtually every other diet out there, and its power to rejuvenate your life and cure your health issues is unparalleled.

And yes, health span is impacted by more than just improving physical health. When you awaken in the morning, reflect for a moment on your sense of purpose for your day ahead. What can you do today, be it small or large, to make your world a better place? A positive outlook is one of the real keys to health and happiness throughout your life. The practice of gratitude or optimism, and acts of kindness, nurturing, and caring will shift the balance of your brain-heart connection away from stress, and towards relaxation and healing.

> "Your time is limited; so don't waste it living someone else's life. Don't let the noise of others' opinions drown out your own inner voice. And most important, have the courage to follow your heart and intuition. They somehow already know what you truly want to become."
> –Steve Jobs

For the rest of your life, you will never be younger than you are right now; so you have no time to waste. At the end of one of Joan's presentations on diet, a gracious elderly gentleman in the audience raised his hand and asked in a worried tone, "Is it too late for me?" Joan replied, "Never, it is never too late. Start today, and use our book as your daily guide to your new health and wellness program." We have learned that when we eat, exercise and rest the way our ancient ancestors did, and remind ourselves to be optimistic and grateful, we can be happy and relaxed, yet focused and energized. To us, it's the best way to spend the time of our lives.

Trying to Make a Difference, One Life at a Time

May is a 61-year-old woman who was out caring for her horses on her ranch one afternoon when she developed the sudden onset of headache, with weakness in her right arm and leg and loss of vision on the right side. She was taken to St. Luke's Hospital where she was treated by the neurology team for a blocked artery in her brain. They consulted us in cardiology for some abnormalities noted on her ECG.

Upon further evaluation, we found that May had suffered a heart attack in the past, and now had blockages in her heart that required we place 2 stents in her coronary arteries. By the time we sent her home from the hospital, she was understandably depressed. One day she thought she was a healthy, middle-aged, active woman, and a few days later she was dealing with repercussions of both a stroke and heart attack. I told her that if she kept on smoking, the cigarettes would probably kill her. I asked her, "Do you have a strategy in mind that you think might get you to stop smoking?" May answered, "Yep. Death."

She wasn't sure life was worth living anymore. I reminded her how much she enjoyed her horses, and how her family loved her deeply. I promised her that things would get better if she would just take things one day at a time and do her best to follow the prescribed regimen of medications, exercise, diet and stay away from tobacco. Six weeks later when she came in for an office visit, I barely recognized her. She was cheerful and vibrant, as she excitedly told me about how one of her mares recently delivered a beautiful little filly. May was using an electronic cigarette but hadn't smoked a single real cigarette; she was eating only healthy food, and getting her daily exercise. She complained a bit about missing the tobacco cigarettes and greasy, junky fast food, but admitted that she was feeling and looking better than she had in years; even her numbness and vision had improved dramatically. As we were wrapping up the visit, I told her, "May I am so proud of you." She smiled at me, and her eyes welled up with tears as she gave me an appreciative embrace.

This experience with May reminded me of a classic fable about a man who was walking down a storm-ravaged section of a sandy beach the morning after a hurricane. He came across a young girl who was picking up starfish that were stranded high and dry on the sand and throwing them, one-by-one, back into the ocean. When the man asked what she was doing, she said he was saving the starfish. To which the man replied, "Young lady, there are untold numbers of stranded starfish dying along these shores, you throwing a few back into the sea isn't going to make any difference." The girl looked up at the man, paused for a moment and then looked back down, bent over and picked up another starfish and threw it gently back into the water. Then the girl turned to the man and said earnestly, "Made a difference for that one."

As a physician and dietitian, we sometimes we get frustrated that most of the people whom we advise to quit smoking and improve their diet and lifestyle don't seem to be able to make it happen. But, I can tell you that to see May thriving and happy again and her grateful hug were more rewarding to me than any monetary payment I could have ever received from her. In our line of work, we make a difference one person at a time. We know this program will work for you, too, whatever your issues are.

CHAPTER 26

The 10 Commandments for Health, Happiness, and a Sexy Waist*

1. Pick a protein morning, noon, and night. Be sure to eat breakfast every morning.

2. Pick at least 2 colors (vegetables and fruits) morning, noon, and night.

3. Drink water, 6 to 8 glasses daily (48 to 64 ounces). Other healthy beverages include: sparkling water, low-sodium V8® juice, skim milk, coconut milk, coffee, and tea. NO sweet beverages (no sweeteners, either natural or artificial).

4. Do not eat or drink anything with added sugar. Also avoid grains; especially shun anything made with wheat, even whole wheat. If you are near your ideal weight, 1 daily serving of whole grain wild rice, quinoa, steel-cut oats, or pearled barley is acceptable.

5. Adopt a pet; a dog that needs daily walking is perfect.

6. Drink in moderation. Not more than 1 or 2 alcoholic drinks daily.

7. Exercise 30 to 50 minutes most days. Shoot for not less than 150 minutes of at least moderate exercise per week. Include weight lifting at least 20 to 30 minutes, 2 or 3 times weekly.

8. Sleep 7½ to 9 hours nightly.

9. Take supplements of omega-3 (1,000 to 1,500 mg of EPA + DHA daily), and vitamin D_3 (2,000 IU daily).

10. Tap into the Power of Love. Put your family first. Commit long-term to your partner/ significant other. Try to stay close, emotionally and physically, to your parents, children, grandparents, and siblings. Build and maintain a social network that supports healthy behaviors such as exercise. Cultivate your spirituality and attend a faith-based service about once per week; denomination does not matter, whatever resonates best with your soul. Even a yoga class can count as spirituality time.

*No tobacco allowed.

Wellness Videos for Inspiration

Make it a point to watch these 3 short videos. They will touch your heart and give you fresh new insights about the power of diet and exercise. Drs. Terry and Mike are both compelling entertainers, to boot.

Google this: Terry Wahl's TED talk (http://www.youtube.com/watch?v=KLjgBLwH3Wc). This is a fascinating 15-minute presentation by Dr. Terry Wahls. She was disabled and dying from progressive multiple sclerosis (MS), despite being treated with all the latest chemotherapeutic regimens.

So, Dr. Wahls took matters into her own hands and learned everything she could about diet. She began following a very strict hunter-gatherer, anti-inflammatory diet based in part upon papers we have published on these topics. She responded dramatically well to this natural and colorful diet. Since her miraculous recovery, she has been testing the diet on other people with advanced MS. She recently presented her breathtaking results at a major neuroscience national meeting. Her diet plan involves eating 3 cups per day of brightly colored fruits and vegetables, 3 cups of leafy greens, and 3 cups of sulfur-containing vegetables, like broccoli, cauliflower, kale, Brussels sprouts, onions, etc. Also, her diet includes seafood, oily fish like wild salmon, and trout, along with game meats and grass-fed beef.

Another must-see video is also on YouTube, entitled *23 and ½ Hours: What Is the Single Best Thing We Can Do for Our Health?* (http://youtube/aUaInS6HIGo). This creative and mesmerizing 8-minute video by Dr. Mike Evans makes a compelling case for daily exercise as the single best thing we can do for our health. Just 30 minutes of walking per day lowers the risk of Alzheimer's by 50 percent, lessens arthritis pain by 47 percent, reduces chances of developing diabetes by 58 percent, lowers anxiety and depression by 48 percent, reduces risk of early death by 23 percent and is the best therapy for reducing fatigue and improving quality of life. Dr. Mike concludes by asking, "Can you limit your sitting and sleeping to just 23 and ½ hours daily?"

Finally, watch my TEDx Talk: *Run for Your Life... at a Comfortable Pace, and Not Too Far: James O'Keefe at TEDxUMKC.* During it I tell stories to explain how and why years to decades of extreme exercise like marathon running can cause cardiovascular problems. In the video I describe healthier exercise patterns for conferring longevity with vitality.

APPENDIX

Additional Information

We are committed to being your trusted and cutting-edge source of cardiovascular and healthful information. We offer the following resources to our patients and public:

- Blog and Newsletter: "From the Heart" and "For the Heart" featuring diet, lifestyle, and health articles written by Joan and me. http://cardionutrition.wordpress.com/author/cardiotabs/

- Free consumer- and clinician-oriented webinars on current health and nutrition topics. Recent examples include: Healthy Strategies to Help Control Your Cholesterol, Diabetes Health, and Dietary Tips to Reduce Your Risk of Developing Cancer.

- E-newsletters featuring relevant consumer health and nutrition information.

- Connect with us:

  Blog and newsletter
  http://cardionutrition.wordpress.com/author/cardiotabs/

  Facebook
  https://www.facebook.com/CardioTabs?fref=ts

- Contact Dr. James O'Keefe or Joan O'Keefe at: www.cardiotabs.com

AUTHORS

James H. O'Keefe, MD, is a cardiologist, and Director of the Charles and Barbara Duboc Cardio Health & Wellness Center at Saint Luke's Mid America Heart Institute. He is also Professor of Medicine at the University of Missouri-Kansas City. His postgraduate training included a cardiology fellowship at Mayo Clinic in Rochester, Minnesota. Dr. O'Keefe is board-certified in Cardiology, Internal Medicine, Nuclear Cardiology, Lipidology, and Cardiac CT Imaging. He is consistently ranked among the 'Top Doctor' lists regionally and nationally. Dr. O'Keefe has contributed more than 250 articles to the medical literature and has authored best seller cardiovascular books for health professionals including: *The Complete Guide to ECGs, Dyslipidemia Essentials*, and *Diabetes Essentials*. He lectures extensively on the role of therapeutic lifestyle changes and drug therapy in cardiovascular risk reduction. He is actively involved in patient care and research. Dr. O'Keefe is the founder of CardioTabs, a nutriceutical company.

Joan O. O'Keefe, RD, was raised in the San Francisco Bay area and received her training to become a Registered Dietitian at the Mayo Clinic in Rochester, MN. She does nutrition counseling focusing on weight loss, optimum health, and improved athletic performance in adults, teens, and kids. She is passionately engaged in teaching others about the nutrition and often speaks to schools, teams, families, men's and women's organizations, and professional groups. Joan and her husband James coauthored the best seller, *The Forever Young Diet & Lifestyle*. She is the mother of 4 children as well as the Chief Executive Officer of CardioTabs, a cardiac nutriceutical company.

INDEX